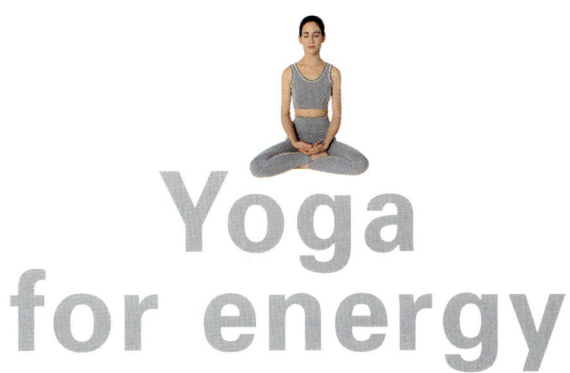

Yoga
for energy

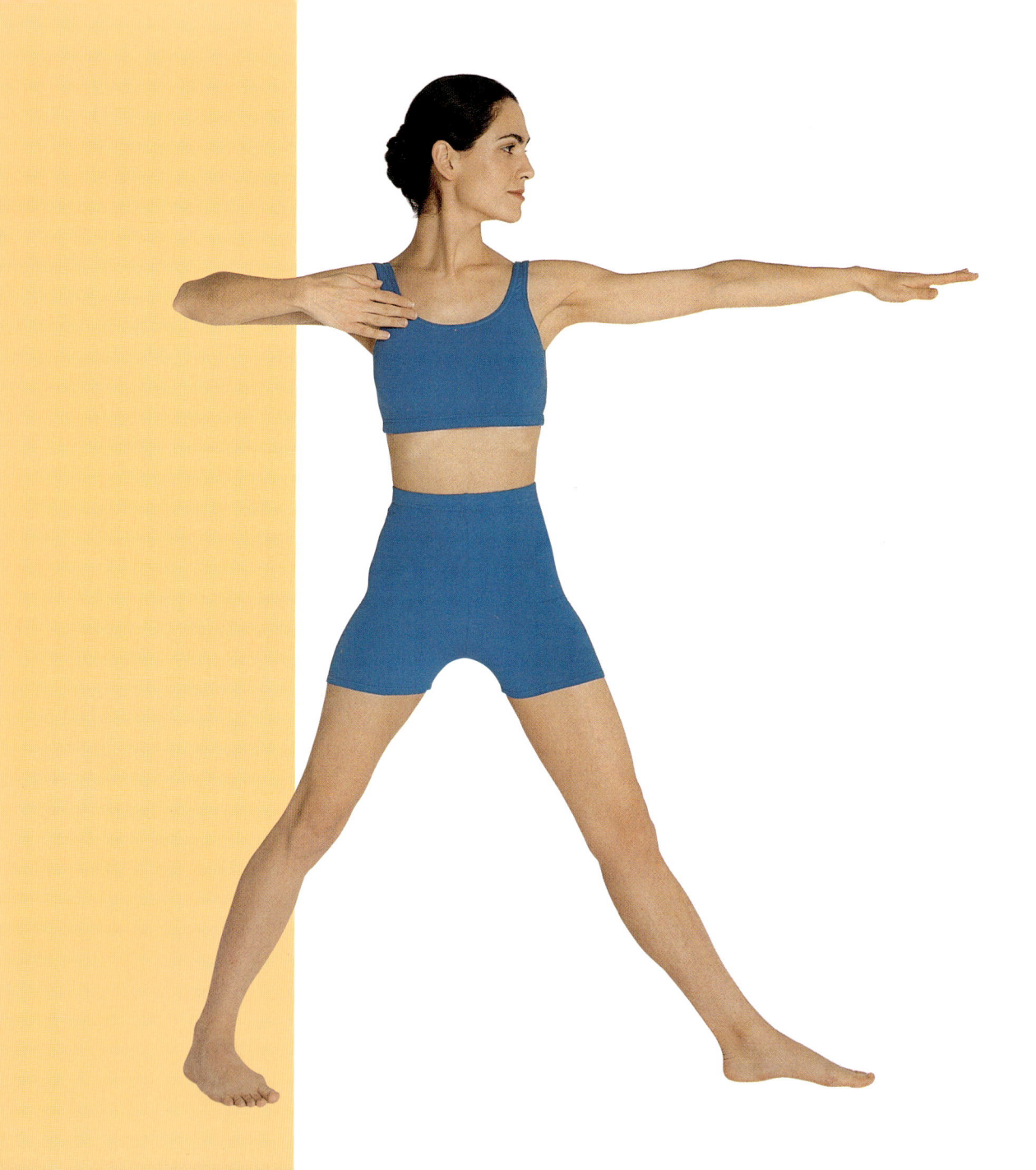

naturally ...

Yoga for energy

Alistair Livingstone

DUNCAN BAIRD PUBLISHERS
LONDON

With gratitude to all my teachers and fellow students

Yoga for energy
Alistair Livingstone

First published in the United Kingdom and Ireland in 2000 by
Duncan Baird Publishers Ltd
Sixth Floor, Castle House
75–76 Wells Street
London W1P 3RE

Conceived, created and designed by Duncan Baird Publishers

Copyright © Duncan Baird Publishers 2000
Text copyright © Duncan Baird Publishers 2000
Commissioned photography copyright © Duncan Baird Publishers 2000

All rights reserved. No part of this book may be reproduced or transmitted in any form or by any means, electronic or mechanical, including photocopying, recording, or by any information-storage or retrieval system now known or hereafter invented without the prior permission in writing of the publisher.

Managing Editor: Judy Dean
Editor: Kesta Desmond
Managing Designer: Manisha Patel
Designer: Rachel Goldsmith
Illustrator: Halli Verrinder
Commissioned photography: Matthew Ward

British Library Cataloguing-in-Publication Data:
A catalogue record for this book is available from the British Library

10 9 8 7 6 5 4 3 2 1

ISBN: 1-900131-74-9

Typeset in Rotis Sans Serif and Univers
Colour reproduction by Colourscan, Singapore
Printed by Imago, Singapore

Note on abbreviations
BCE (Before the Common Era) is the equivalent of BC.
CE (Common Era) is the equivalent of AD.

Publisher's note
Before following any advice or practice suggested in this book, it is recommended that you consult your doctor as to its suitability, especially if you suffer from any health problems or special conditions. The publishers, the author and the photographers cannot accept responsibility for any injuries or damage incurred as a result of following the exercises in this book, or using any of the therapeutic methods described or mentioned here.

Contents

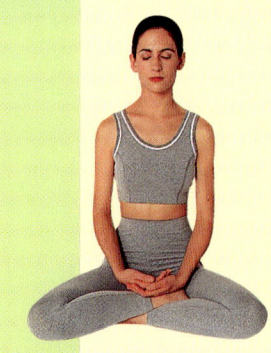

Introduction 6

What is yoga? 9
Paths to yoga 10
Subtle anatomy 12
Moving to stillness 14

Preparing the self 17
Relaxation posture 18
Simply sitting 20
Standing tall 22
Yoga breathing 24
Warming the body 26

Enhancing the energy flow 29
Arm stretches 30
Forward bend 32
The cat 34
Downward-facing dog 36
Pose of the child 38
Leg lift 40
The cobra 42
The thunderbolt 44

The butterfly 46
Easy spinal twist 48
The half-moon 50
The archer 52
The bridge 54
The plank 56
Half-shoulder stand 58
The fish 60

Yoga all day 63
Morning stretch 64
Yoga at work 66
Evening practice 68
Bedtime relaxation 70

Index 72
Acknowledgments 72

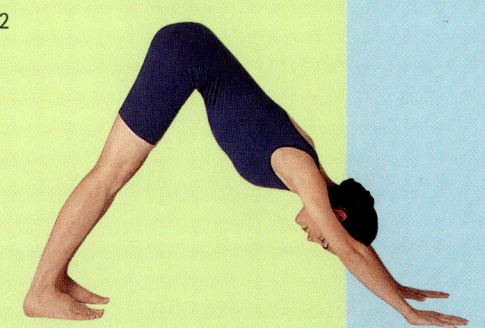

Introduction

Suddenly it seems as if everyone is practising some form of yoga. This very ancient form of personal integration is increasingly recognized as a way to improve the appearance of the body, stay fit and prevent or treat health problems. The best way to learn yoga is from an experienced teacher or yoga therapist who will encourage you to work slowly and systematically toward the classic postures and will modify practices specifically for your body and needs. *Yoga for Energy* introduces a diverse range of yoga practices that you can do by yourself throughout the day, at home or at work, without the guidance of an instructor. The postures, breathing practices and relaxation techniques found in this book will help you to still your mind, revitalize your body and restore your energy levels. Many practices are modified for people who are new to yoga, so that you can perform them easily and safely. Enjoy your yoga practice!

Hari om tat sat

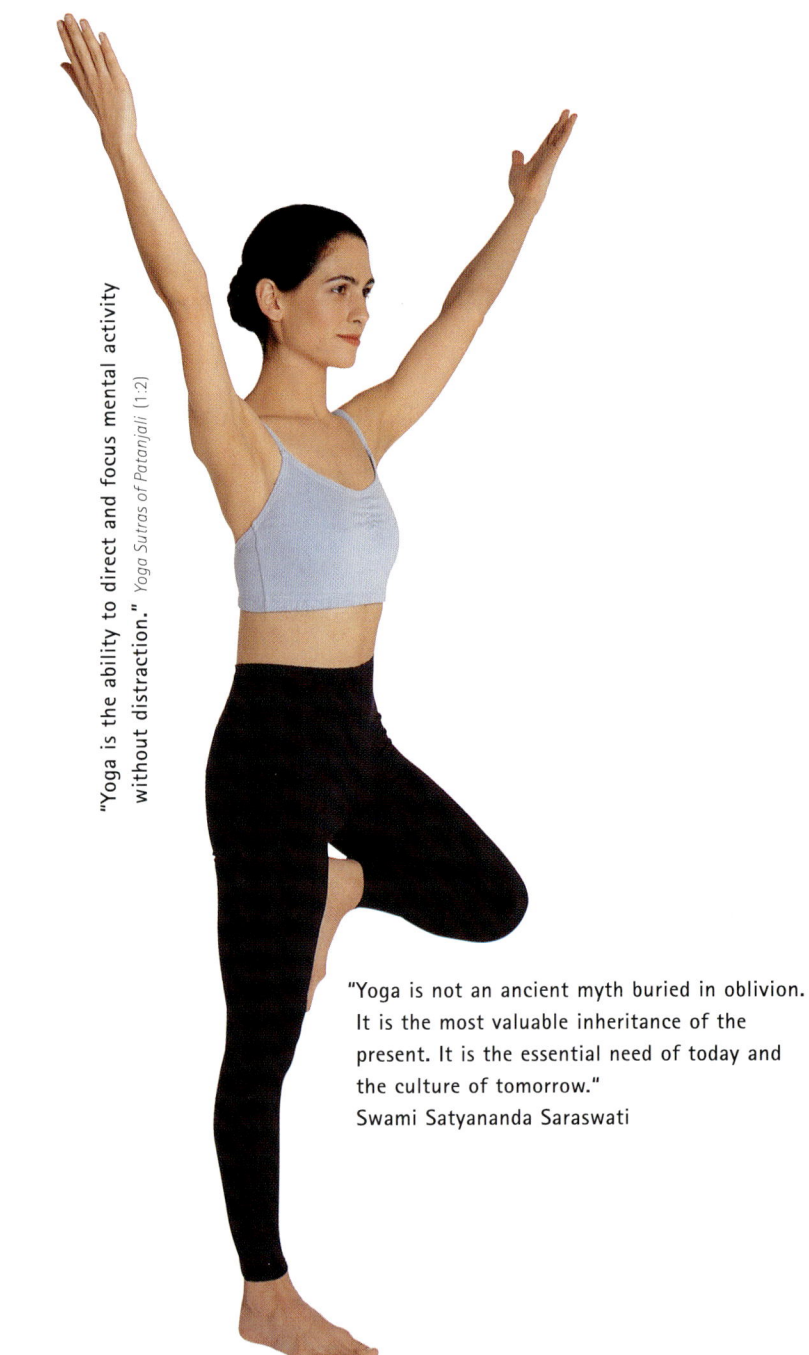

"Yoga is the ability to direct and focus mental activity without distraction." *Yoga Sutras of Patanjali* (1:2)

"Yoga is not an ancient myth buried in oblivion. It is the most valuable inheritance of the present. It is the essential need of today and the culture of tomorrow."
Swami Satyananda Saraswati

chapter one
What is yoga?

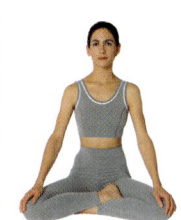

Yoga is a way of integrating the mind, body and spirit, leading you to a healthier and more fulfilled life.

The earliest archaeological evidence of yoga dates from about 3000BCE in the Indus Valley, where statues depicting deities in yoga postures have been found. Yoga philosophy appears in texts such as the *Yoga Sutras of Patanjali*, dating from the 3rd century BCE, and in the *Bhagavad Gita*, from around the 6th century BCE.

The Sanskrit word for yoga is *yuj*, meaning "to join" or "union". At the highest level this implies uniting individual consciousness with universal consciousness.

Paths to yoga
posture, breathing and meditation

There are many different paths to yoga. Four of the main ones are: Karma yoga (the yoga of action), Bhakti yoga (the yoga of devotion), Jnana yoga (the yoga of knowledge) and Raja yoga. The fourth form, Raja yoga (often called the "royal road"), can be considered the mastery of mind and body in order to release the higher nature. Hatha yoga is widely practised in the West and is a sub-division of Raja yoga. Hatha yoga includes the practice of posture (*asana*), breathing (*pranayama*), meditation (*dhyana*) and cleansing practices (*shatkarmas*).

The various postures and breathing techniques that form the basis of the modern practice of Hatha yoga are contained in the classic 8th- and 9th-century text, *Hatha Yoga Pradipika*.

The *asanas* work on stretching and toning the muscles and skeletal framework of the body, as well as conditioning the organs and the nervous system. *Pranayama* practices calm the mind and revitalize the entire being. Relaxation and *dhyana* bring increased concentration and clarity. The cleansing practices of Hatha yoga, known as *shatkarmas* or *kriyas*, are very powerful and should only be learnt from a teacher.

Regularly practising yoga helps to restore balance and harmony in the body and mind, removes toxins from the body and releases vast resources of untapped energy.

"Prior to everything, asana **is spoken of as the first part of Hatha yoga."** *Hatha Yoga Pradipika* (1:17)

Subtle anatomy
chakras and *nadis*

Western medicine tends to view the body as a collection of replaceable parts, many of which can be treated in isolation from one another. Other traditions view the body in a more holistic way, recognizing an essential inner energy, known as "life-force energy" or "vital force". In yoga teaching this energy is known as *prana*; when the balance of *prana* is disrupted, the result is illness. In yoga tradition the body has a system of chakras and *nadis* (channels) that generate and regulate *prana*. There are seven chakras on the midline of the body and many *nadis* through which *prana* flows.

> "The removal of impurities allows the body to function more efficiently." *Yoga Sutras of Patanjali* (2:43)

Although chakras cannot be seen physically, they do have a relationship with the major physical organs in the body. They are positioned along the line of the spine. Many healers describe them as "spinning wheels of energy" and they are often represented by sound and colour. The chakras are connected by three main *nadis*: *ida*, which passes by the left nostril; *pingala*, which passes by the right nostril; and *sushumna*, which runs up the middle of the spine. *Pranayama* and *asana* practice balances the flow of *prana*. Concentrating on certain chakras during *asana* practice can enhance the benefits of a posture.

- Crown chakra – *sahasrara*
- Third-eye chakra – *ajna*
- Throat chakra – *vishuddhi*
- Heart chakra – *anahata*
- Solar-plexus chakra – *manipura*
- Sacral chakra – *swadhisthana*
- Base chakra – *muladhara*

- Left side – *ida*
- Right side – *pingala*
- Centre – *sushumna*

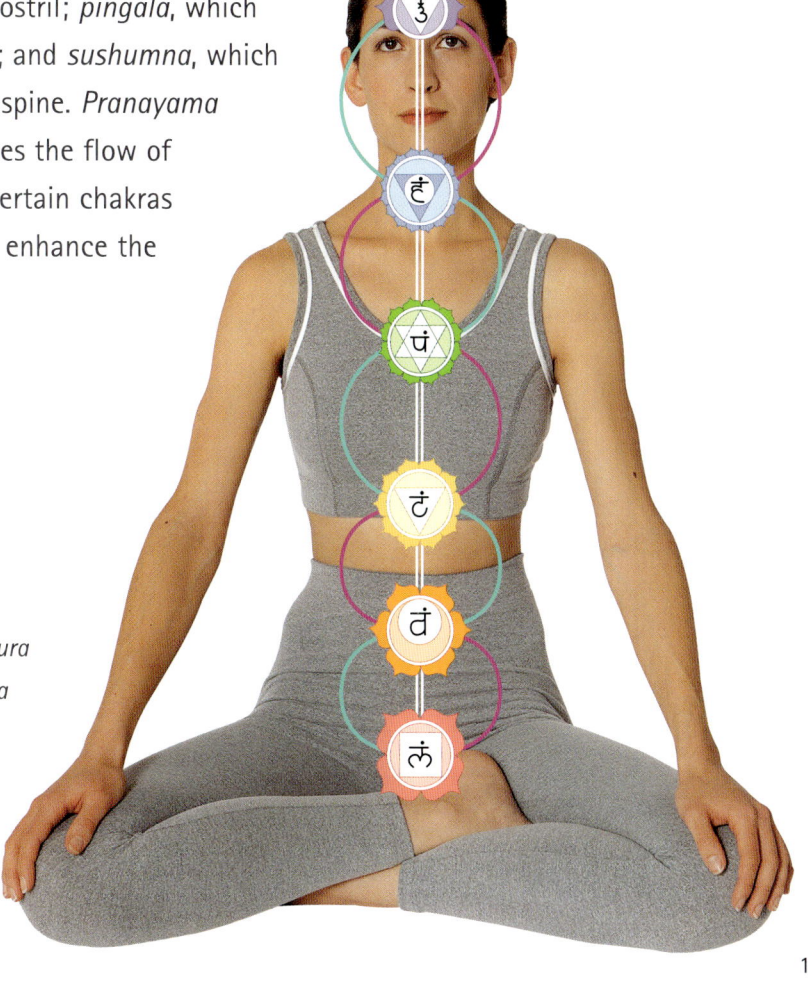

Moving to stillness
making contact with *purusa*

Most of us live in a stressful environment. Some stress is useful – it drives us to meet our goals. Most of us, however, add unnecessarily to the stress in our lives; we often rush to and from work on busy transport systems, we carry too many bags, and we sit and stand in ways that make the body stiff and misaligned. Whether we are at work or at home, we spend much time sitting in front of a computer or television screen. All of these things sap our energy. Although it is impossible to banish stress entirely, we can learn ways to manage it. A main aim of yoga is to find a place of spiritual stillness from which to respond to the world: achieving stillness in postures and mastering your breath are vital steps toward this.

People often start to practise yoga because they wish to change something in their lives: to feel more healthy, be more positive, think more clearly, be calmer or have more energy. This impetus for change ultimately comes from a place deep within us that yearns to be quiet and content and free from judgment and blame. In Sanskrit this spiritual place is known as *purusa*.

Yoga is not about striving for the impossible – that is, attempting to achieve incredibly complex postures before you are ready. It is about working within your limits and developing a personal practice that brings you into contact with your internal energy flow and self-awareness. By learning to direct energy through the use of breath, the body, mind and emotions will come into harmony. This in turn leads you to a place of quiet and stillness, where decisions can be made with clarity and insight. Once you make contact with this place of stillness, you will notice that stressful parts of your life become more manageable. Make a commitment to live your life responsibly, fully experiencing each moment from a quiet place of understanding: this is yoga.

> "The mind can reach the state of yoga through tireless endeavour and non-attachment." *Yoga Sutras of Patanjali* (1:12)

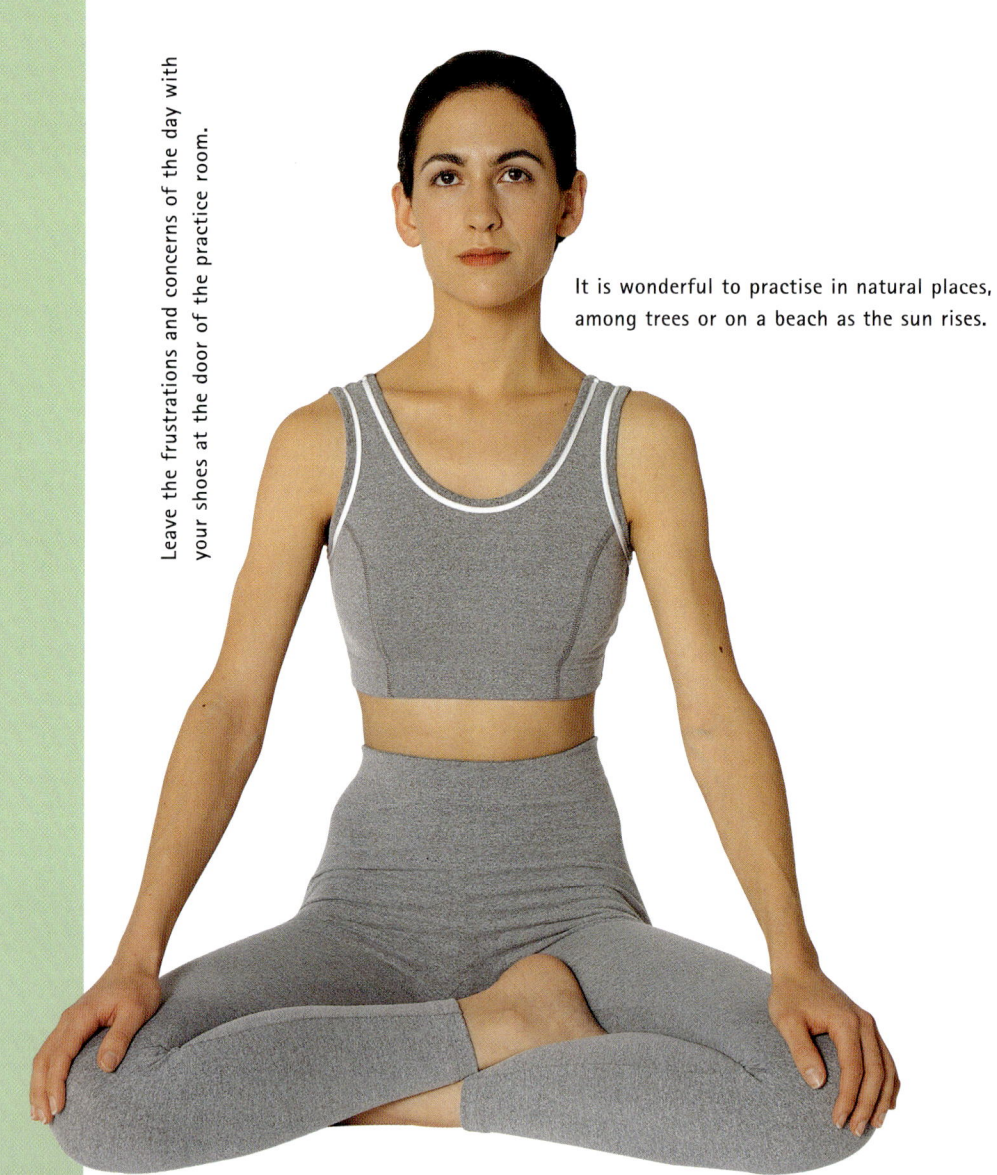

Leave the frustrations and concerns of the day with your shoes at the door of the practice room.

It is wonderful to practise in natural places, among trees or on a beach as the sun rises.

chapter two
Preparing the self

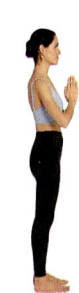

Wherever possible, practise yoga in bare feet in a warm, ventilated space. Wear clothes that are loose and comfortable.

This chapter serves as a gentle introduction to some important, basic yoga postures. Each posture can be explored in depth: try to work on developing your concentration and breathing in each one. Remember that yoga should be fun – never struggle or do anything painful, and try to avoid eating for a few hours before you practise.

Some people like to use a special mat, light a candle and incense and even play gentle music when they do yoga, but this is entirely up to you. Most importantly, you need to feel at ease with yourself and your surroundings.

Relaxation posture

Shavasana, the corpse pose

Shavasana is one of the most important *asanas* in yoga. You can use it to centre yourself at the start of a yoga practice, and at the end as a final relaxation. You can also use it as a resting posture between more dynamic *asanas*. It is called the corpse pose because it requires you to lie perfectly still, and to slow your breath. This helps the mind to become quiet. Once you have mastered this posture, you can use it to relax at any time.

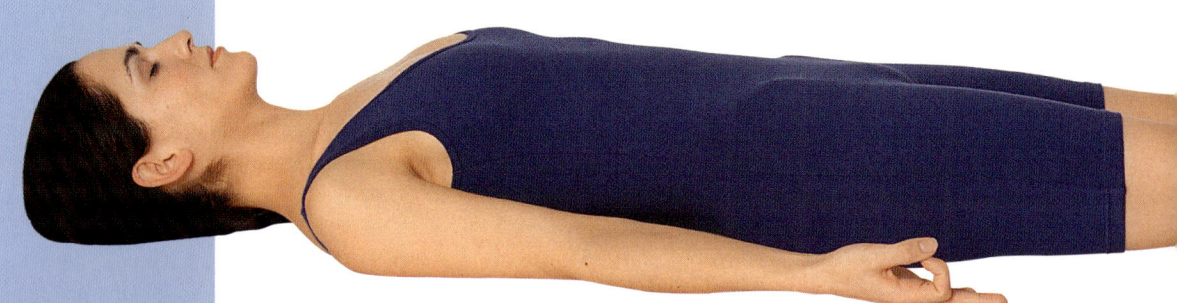

Lie down on your back, preferably on a blanket or a mat. You may need a folded blanket underneath your head for comfort. Visualize an imaginary line running from the top of your head to between your feet. Your body should be lying equally on either side of this line. Your hands should be about 6 in (15 cm) away from your body with your palms facing upward. Your feet should be 12–16 in (30–40 cm) apart. Lift your pelvis and lightly reposition it to let the spine lengthen. Allow each vertebra to relax and sink into the floor. Check that your head is straight and not to one side.

Now relax completely, knowing that your body and being are supported. Concentrate on the tip of your nose and focus on the breath as it enters and leaves the nostrils. Follow the breath up your nose then down into your throat and lungs. Imagine that you are floating above yourself, observing your body lying on the floor. Breathe "into" any points of tension, allowing them to dissolve. Finally, bring your awareness back to the tip of your nose. Think to yourself: "I know I am breathing in, I know I am breathing out."

If you have lower-back problems, you can make this pose more comfortable by putting a bolster or cushion under your knees.

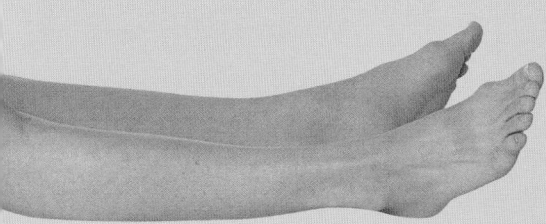

Simply sitting

Dandasana, the staff pose

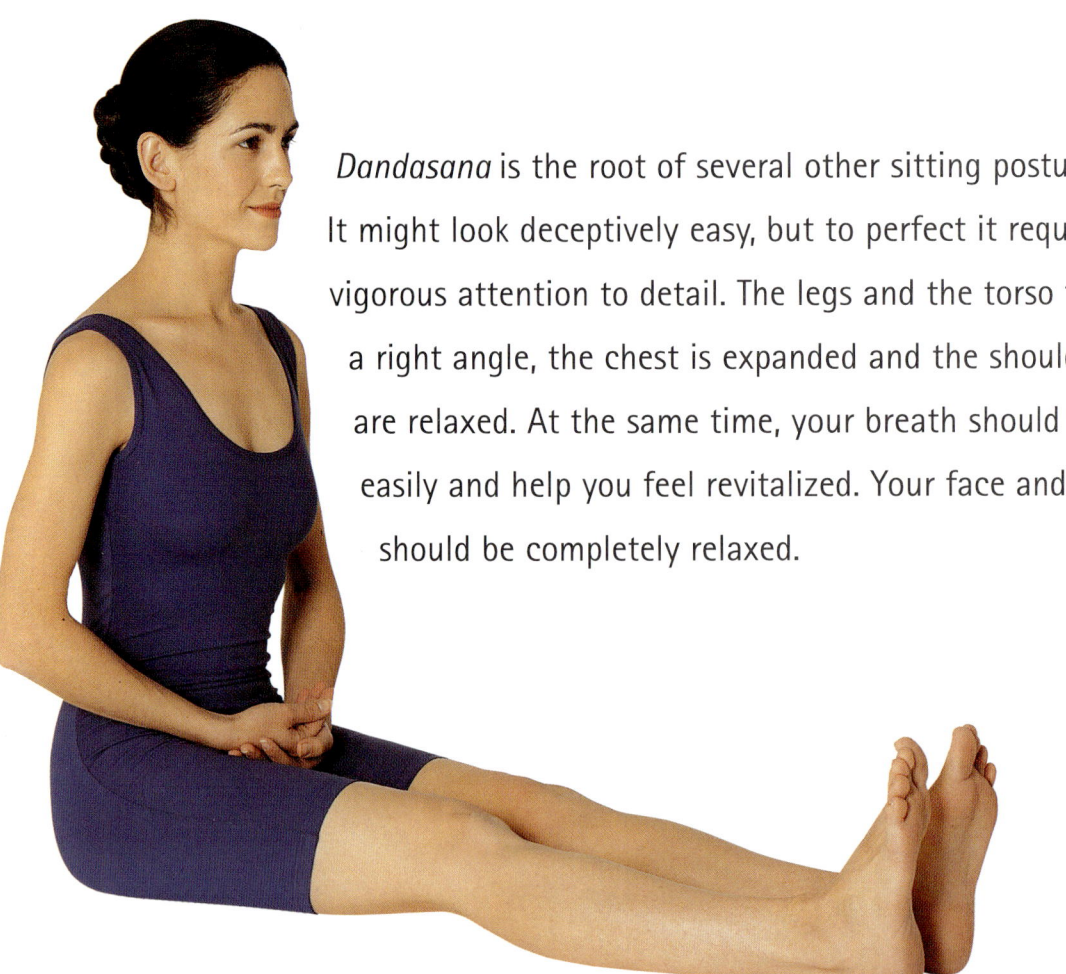

Dandasana is the root of several other sitting postures. It might look deceptively easy, but to perfect it requires vigorous attention to detail. The legs and the torso form a right angle, the chest is expanded and the shoulders are relaxed. At the same time, your breath should flow easily and help you feel revitalized. Your face and jaw should be completely relaxed.

Sit with your legs stretched out in front of you. Place your hands on the floor by your hips, either with your palms flat or on your fingertips. Supporting yourself on your hands, lift your hips off the floor and move the base of your spine back a little before lowering yourself again. You should now feel solidly rooted to the ground. Tighten your knees and stretch your heels away from you, with your ankles gently flexed and your toes pointing upward.

Press down on your fingertips and breathe in. Extend your spine upward, lengthen your lower back and imagine the top of your head is held on a fine thread. Open your chest area and lift your shoulders up and back. Breathe out. Let your eye muscles relax so that your focus is soft (or close your eyes). Now relax your jaw, cheeks, forehead and scalp. Release any remaining tension on each out-breath.

Raise your arms and make your hands into fists with your thumbs enclosed in your fingers. Breathe in. As you breathe out, flick your fingers outward, stretching them as far as you can. Then bring your fingers to the floor or fold your hands in your lap and return your awareness to your breathing.

Learning to sit without discomfort is fundamental to good yoga practice.

Standing tall
Tadasana, the mountain pose

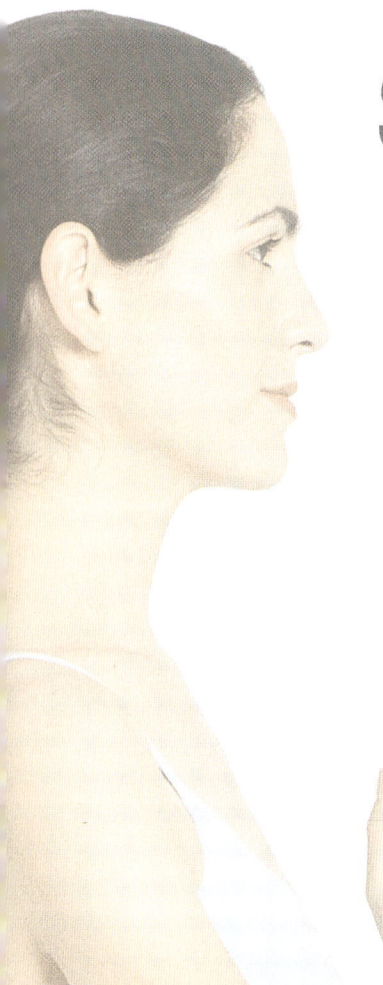

We often overlook the energy-giving potential of everyday postures. Even an apparently simple standing position such as *tadasana* can be invigorating. The mountain pose helps to release tension that builds up imperceptibly in our bodies throughout the day. It may be considered one of the most fundamental *asanas* – the point of departure not just for the other standing postures, but for all yoga postures.

The idea of the mountain suggests stillness, strength and steadfastness – all crucial elements of yoga practice.

Stand with your feet close together, the inside edges parallel and nearly touching. If this is uncomfortable, move them apart slightly. Take your awareness down to the soles of your feet and feel the connection with the ground. Spread your toes. Shift your weight back a little and ensure that your heels are firmly on the floor. Imagine that you have strong roots that reach down from your feet into the earth, enabling you to draw energy up into your body. Visualize the flow of energy up your lower body as you tighten and relax each group of muscles and ligaments in turn: first the ankles, then the calves, knees (you may need to bend them slightly), thighs and hips.

Take a deep breath and, as you exhale, check that your lower limbs are relaxed. Tip your hips forward slightly, while gently pulling the abdominal muscles upward. Move your awareness to your diaphragm, chest and shoulders, and tense and relax each in turn. Take another deep breath in and raise your shoulders toward your ears. On your out-breath allow your shoulders to drop and relax. Imagine a fine thread gently pulling you by the top of the head toward the sky. Inhale, then say "ha" as you let the air out. Finally, bring your hands together in front of your chest in the prayer position, and breathe in and out, not controlling the breath but simply letting it flow.

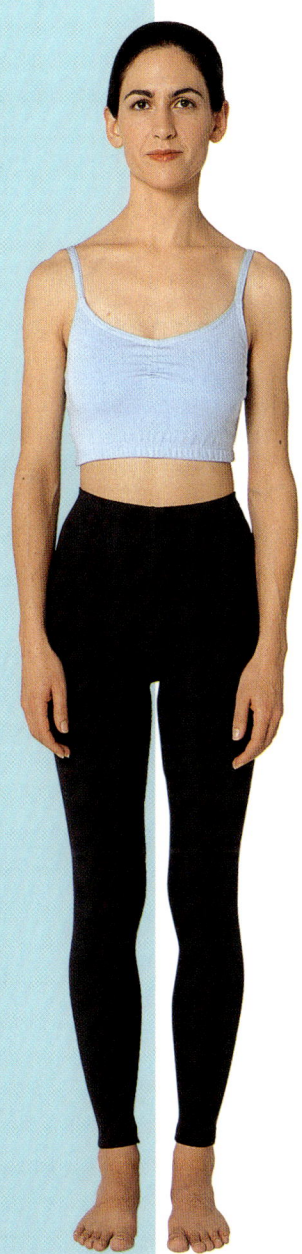

Yoga breathing
Pranayama

The key to yoga lies in the use of the breath. Because breathing is an automatic process, most of the time we are not aware of it and do not breathe to full capacity. *Pranayama* practice focuses awareness on the breath and the ability of pranic energy to revitalize the being. Most movements in *asana* practice are linked to in-breaths and out-breaths. Try to breathe through your nose, synchronizing each breath with the movement of your body.

Prana **means "vital force" or "life-force energy";** ayama **is defined as "expansion".**

Sit in a comfortable cross-legged position, press your palms on the floor and extend your spine upward, opening your chest. Place your palms on your knees.

Then place one hand on your abdomen at the level of the navel and breathe in slowly and deeply, allowing the abdomen to balloon outward. Breathe out slowly, using the abdominal muscles to contract the abdomen and expel all the remaining air. Repeat twice.

Now move both hands to the bottom of the rib cage so that the middle fingertips lie touching one another along the line of the lowest rib. Breathe in, expanding the rib cage as far as possible to the front, back and sides. Notice how far the fingers separate. (Check this again after a few months – you may find your lung capacity has increased.) Repeat twice.

Cross your arms and place your fingertips just below your collarbones. Breathe into the area at the top of the lungs, letting the breath come up as high as possible without straining. Let any tension drop away from your jaw or neck. Repeat twice. Now try to put the 3 actions together: breathe slowly and smoothly into the abdomen, rib cage and the top of the chest in one continuous inhalation. Then release the breath from the body. Repeat up to 5 times.

"Having gained control of the body through asana practice, pranayamas should be practised." *Hatha Yoga Pradipika* (2:1)

Warming the body
Pawanmuktasanas

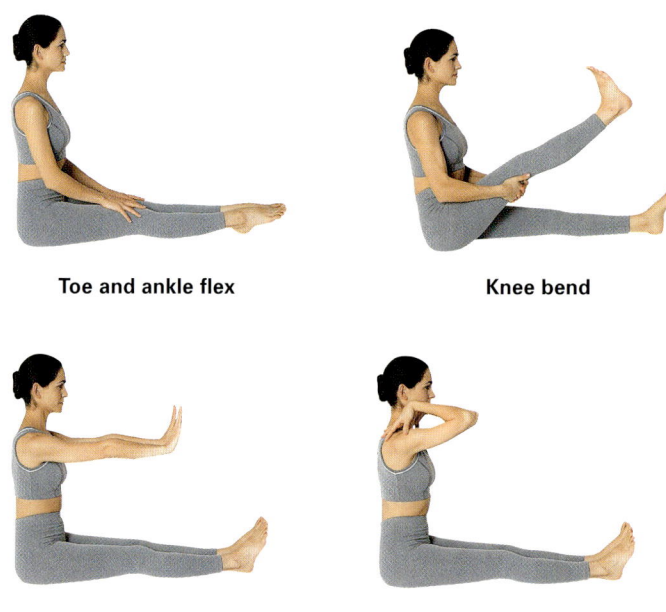

Toe and ankle flex   **Knee bend**

Wrist bend   **Shoulder rotation**

These warm-ups prepare the body for more dynamic postures by releasing energy blockages in joints and muscles. They can also help to alleviate rheumatism and arthritis, and are excellent for people who are advised not to practise more strenuous postures.

You can do these postures at home or at work, sitting on a chair or sitting on the floor – whichever is easier.

Toe and ankle flex Breathe in and curl your toes back toward your body. Breathe out and curl them away. Repeat 5 times. Now do the same with your entire foot.

Knee bend Lift your right leg with both hands under the back of the knee. Breathe in and straighten your leg. Breathe out and bend your leg. Do not let your heel touch the floor. Repeat 5 times and then change legs.

Wrist bend Stretch your arms out in front. Breathe in and bend your hands back at the wrists. Breathe out and extend them forward and down. Repeat 5 times.

Shoulder rotation With your fingertips on the tops of your shoulders, rotate your elbows in a small circle. Make the circle bigger and include the shoulders in the movement. Breathe in as your elbows rise and out as they drop. Repeat 5 times then reverse direction.

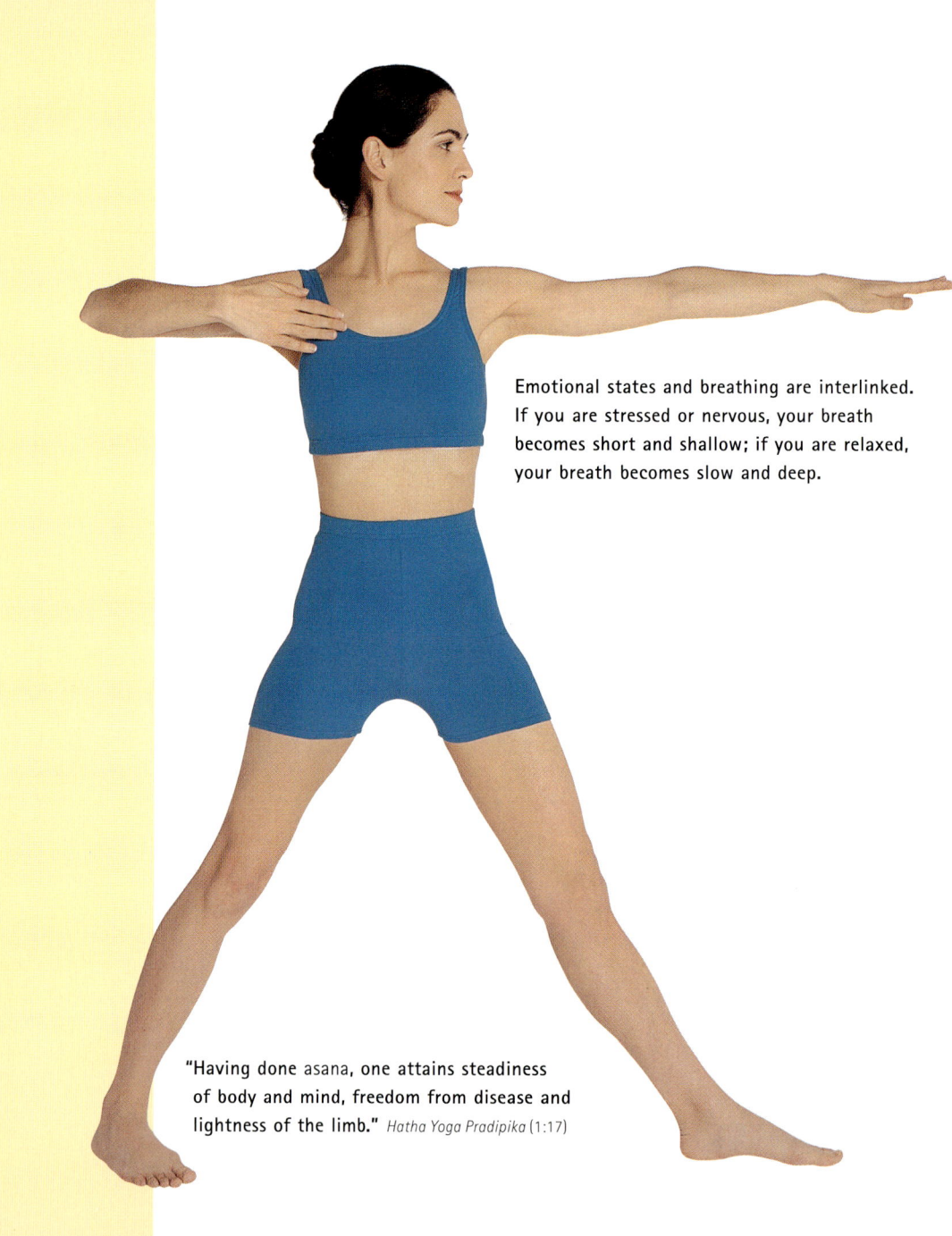

Emotional states and breathing are interlinked. If you are stressed or nervous, your breath becomes short and shallow; if you are relaxed, your breath becomes slow and deep.

"Having done asana, one attains steadiness of body and mind, freedom from disease and lightness of the limb." *Hatha Yoga Pradipika* (1:17)

chapter three

Enhancing the energy flow

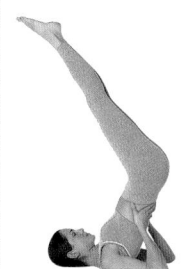

The energizing postures in this chapter can be practised on their own, in small groups or as one long sequence.

The following yoga postures are easily attainable for most people (consult a doctor or yoga teacher if you are in doubt about whether yoga is right for you). Start your practice in a calm frame of mind and try to coordinate your breathing with the movements of your body. If you find this difficult, concentrate on the postures first then focus on your breathing later. Learning to direct your breath within the postures will boost your energy levels and make you better equipped to deal with stressful situations. It will also help to make your yoga practice easier and more enjoyable.

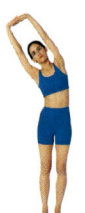

Arm stretches
tiryaka tadasana

❶ Stand with your feet slightly apart, arms at your sides. ❷ Stretch your arms out in front of you. Link your fingers, palms facing in. Breathe in. ❸ Turn your palms out. Breathe out. ❹ Breathe in and raise your arms slowly above your head. Stretch upward with your arms straight and your palms facing the ceiling. ❺ Stretch to the right, extending the left side of your body. Breathe out. ❻ Breathe in and return to centre. ❼ Stretch to the left, extending the right side of your body. Breathe out. Breathe in and return to centre. ❽ Breathe out and lower your arms to your sides. ❾ Stand in the start position for a few moments then repeat the sequence twice more.

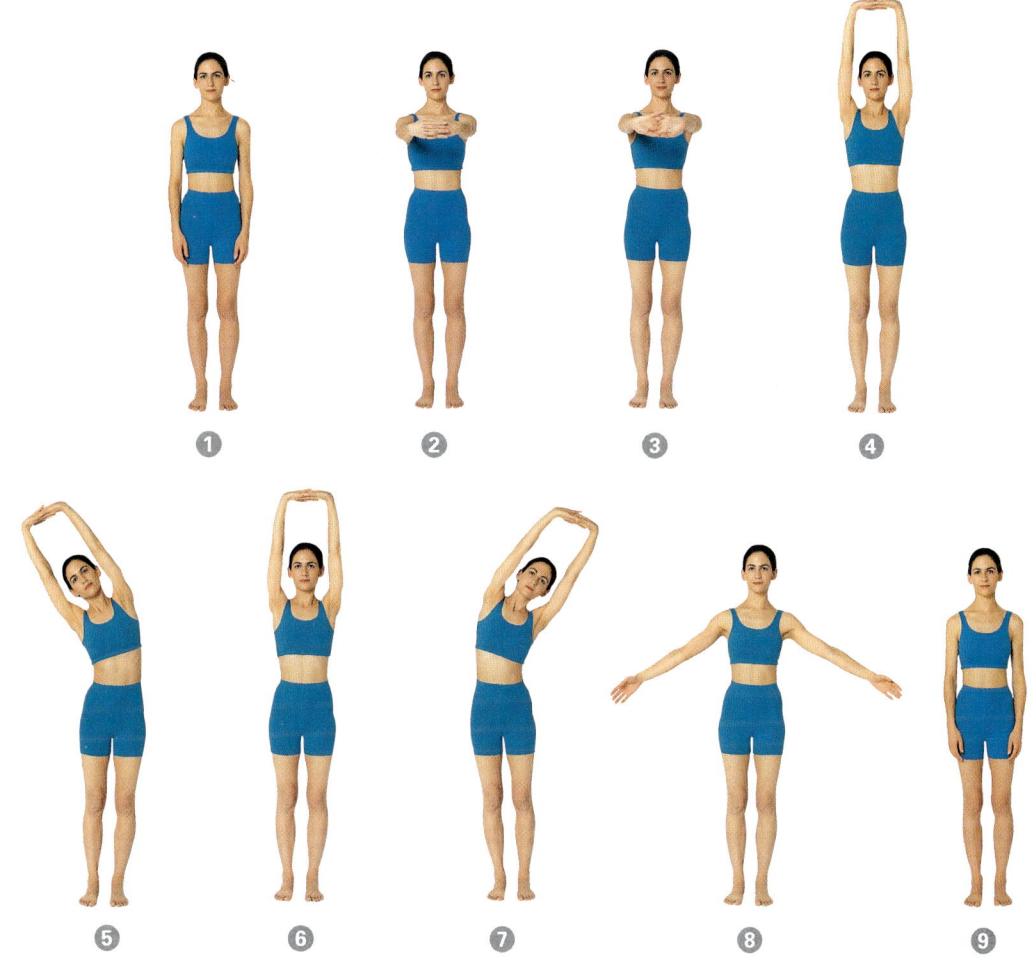

Stretching upward energizes the body, especially when accompanied by yogic breathing. Side stretches keep joints flexible and open the vertebrae laterally. In everyday life the spine is not usually extended in this way.

The movements of these arm stretches signify an ability to move the upper part of our body with the winds of change yet to keep our feet firmly planted on the ground.

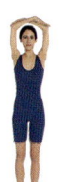

Forward bend
utthanasana

❶ Stand with your feet slightly apart and your hands together in the prayer position. ❷ Breathing in, raise both hands above your head, palms facing. Keep your arms straight and parallel, your fingers pointing up. ❸ Breathing out, fold your arms above your head. Grip your elbows. Breathe in. ❹ Breathing out, bend at your hips and knees as if going to sit down. ❺ Bend forward and lower your palms to the floor. ❻ Breathing in, let your fingers slide over your feet, ankles and the fronts of your legs. Straighten your knees and slowly stand up. ❼ Breathing out, bring your hands back to the prayer position. Repeat the sequence, reversing the clasp of your elbows.

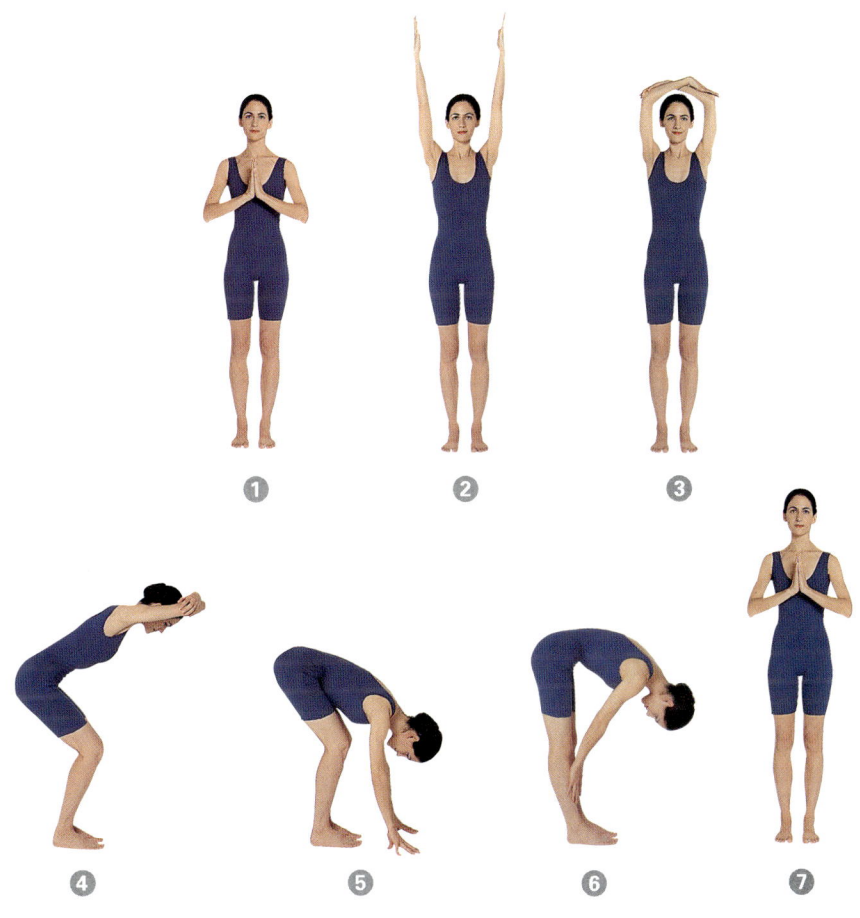

This *asana* sequence makes you feel refreshed and invigorated, and regular practice builds your energy levels so that you don't tire so easily. You should approach this sequence slowly. If you have any lower-back problems or suffer from high blood pressure, consult your doctor or a qualified yoga therapist first.

This sequence tones your back muscles and helps to make your spine more flexible.

The cat
marjari-asana

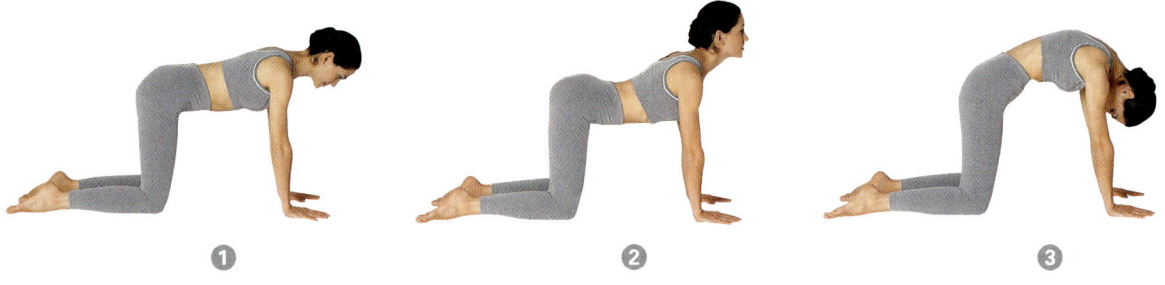

This posture frees the spine and neck, improves the circulation, and stimulates the digestive tract and spinal fluids. It is a useful posture for women who experience menstrual cramps. The Cat posture also teaches you to coordinate your breath with your movements.

When you practise this posture, focus on the eyebrow chakra (ajna) **as you breathe in and on the sacral chakra** (swadhistana) **as you breathe out.**

❶ Start on your hands and knees. Your hands should be directly under your shoulders with your fingers spread out and your middle fingers pointing forward. Your knees should be directly under your hips, with your thighs at right angles to your calves. ❷ As you breathe in, slowly roll your eyes upward and then raise your head, neck and shoulders to follow. Allow your spine to dip and your hips to tilt so that your tailbone points upward. ❸ As you breathe out, pull your abdominal muscles up toward your spine and allow your hips to tilt forward and your head to come down so that your spine curves upward. Repeat this sequence up to 5 times.

Downward-facing dog
adho mukha shvanasana

❶ Start on your hands and knees. Your palms should be shoulders' width apart and your fingers should be spread with your middle fingers pointing forward. Take a moment or two to breathe in and out, then curl your toes under your feet. **❷** Breathing in, let your knees come off the floor – imagine that you are being pulled up into the air by the base of your spine. Keep your knees bent and allow your chest to come close to your thighs. **❸** Breathing out, try to release your heels so that they sink to the floor. Straighten your knees and lift your hips. Relax your neck and shoulders. Keep breathing. Hold the posture for as long as you feel comfortable and steady.

① ② ③

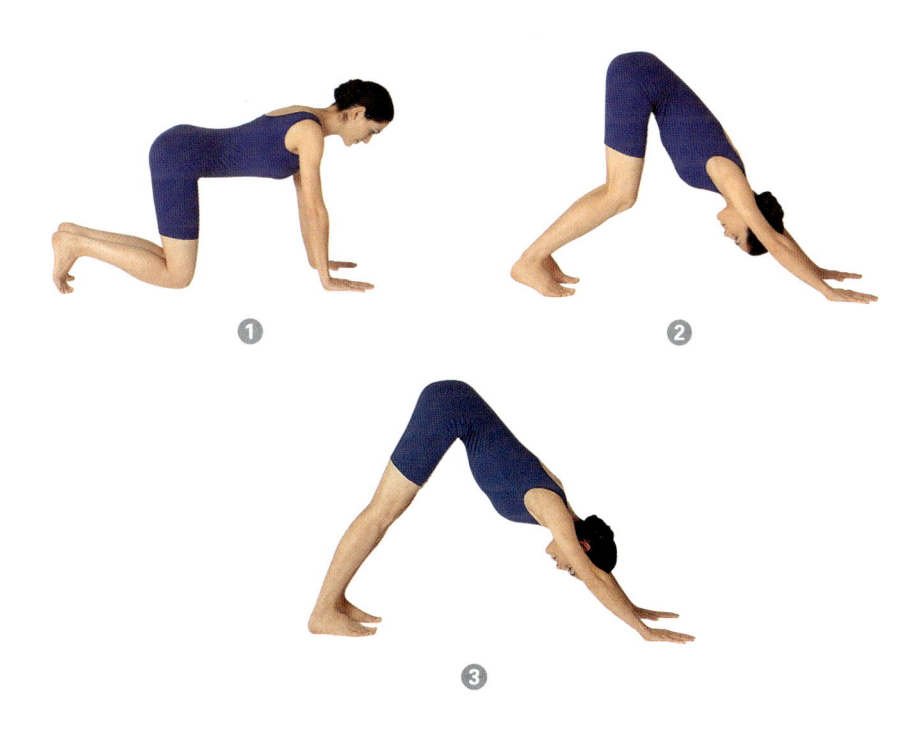

Downward-facing dog strengthens your arm and leg muscles, your spine and the long bones of your arms and legs. It also stimulates the circulation and nerves in the upper back and shoulders. When you practise this posture, focus your attention on the throat chakra (*vishuddhi*).

My wonderful teacher, Swami Ajnananda, always used to remind his students that the Downward-facing dog is a posture in which they could meditate!

Pose of the child
supta shashankasana

❶ Start on your hands and knees. **❷** Push back, sit on your heels and extend your arms. Gently rest your forehead on the floor. Feel the stretch and allow your spine to lengthen. Sink more deeply into the posture with each out-breath. **❸** Make your hands into fists. Slide them back, resting one on top of the other under your forehead. **❹** Sit back on your heels with your palms on your knees. **❺** Breathing in, raise your arms in an arc in front of your body, above your head. Keep your palms facing in and your elbows straight. Breathe out and lower your arms. **❻** Gently lower your forehead to the floor and extend your arms behind you, resting them by your sides.

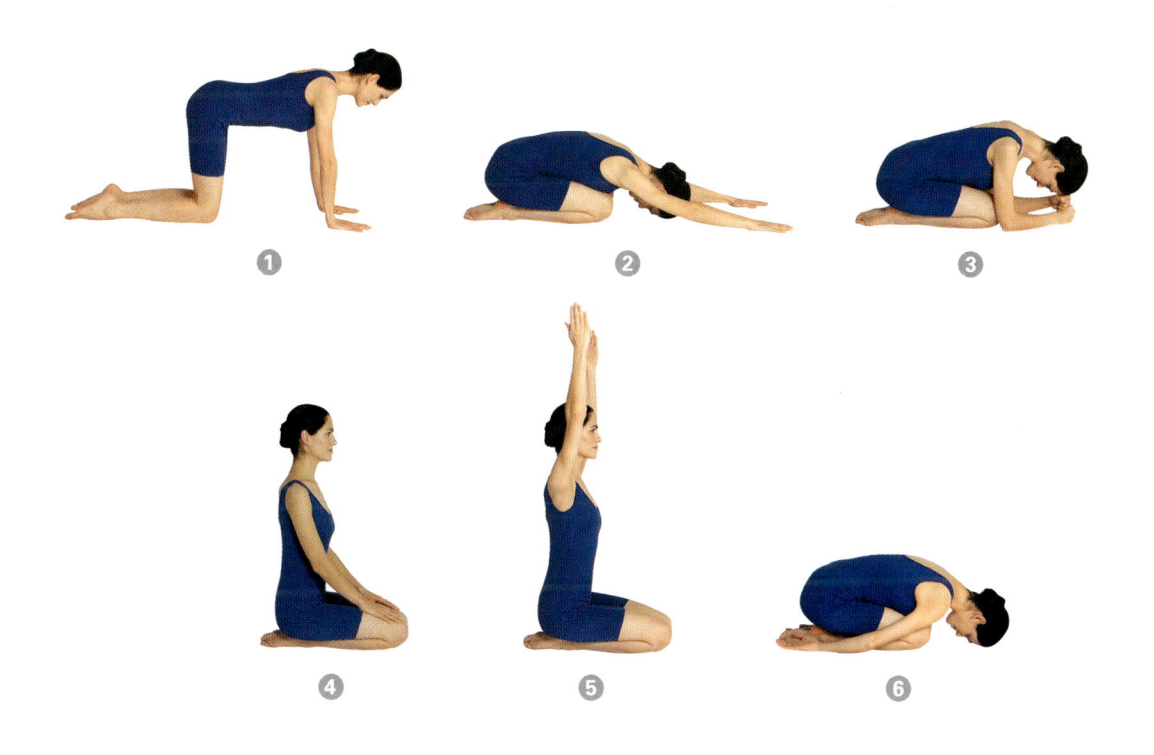

This series relaxes the spinal ligaments and stretches the back muscles. The final posture relieves compression on the intervertebral disks which become compacted when standing. It is a wonderfully relaxing posture.

If you find it difficult to sit back on your heels, try putting a cushion under your buttocks and sit on this. You can even try one under your feet as well.

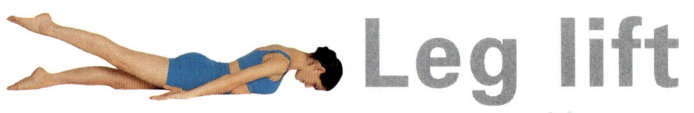

Leg lift
ardha shalabhasana

1 Lie face down and fold your arms in front of you, with one forearm on top of the other. Turn your head to one side and rest it on your arms. Focus on your breath – let it flow naturally. **2** Move your arms to your sides, palms facing upward. Your forehead should rest on the floor. **3** Breathe in and raise your left leg from the hip. Keep the knee straight. Breathe out and gently lower your leg. Repeat up to 5 times. **4** Repeat Step 3 with your right leg. **5** Press down with your arms and raise both legs together. Repeat up to 5 times. Return to Step 1 and rest with your head facing in the opposite direction.

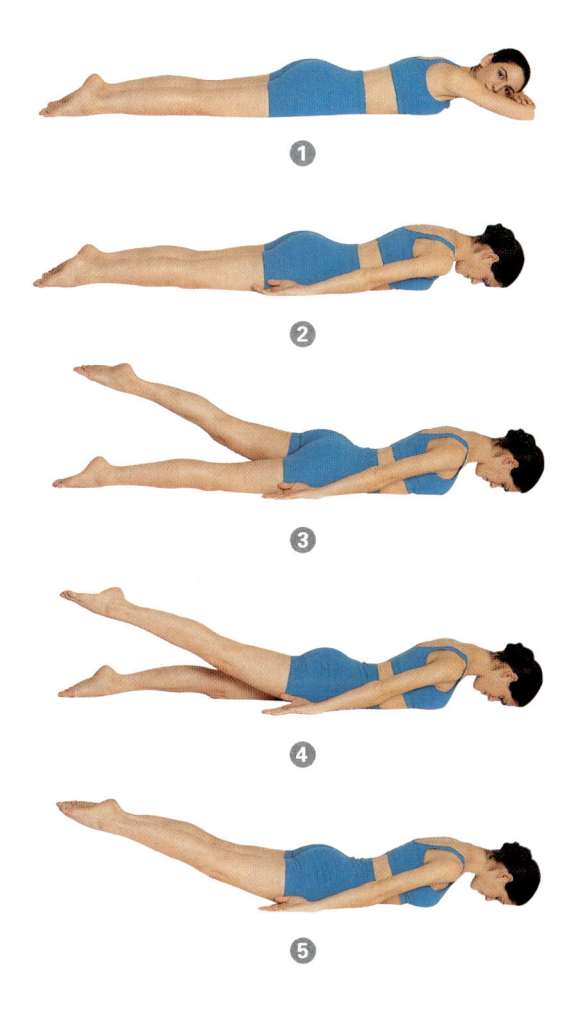

The Leg lift is helpful for beginners as it stimulates the nerves in the lower back and helps to strengthen the back muscles. Synchronizing breath and movement helps to develop concentration. When you practise the Leg lift, focus your attention on the sacral chakra (*swadhisthana*).

Don't attempt to lift both legs together until you are entirely comfortable raising the legs individually.

The cobra
bhujangasana

❶ Lie flat on your stomach with your legs extended and your feet together. Fold your arms and rest your head on them. Relax your leg muscles. **❷** Bring your hands underneath and slightly to the sides of your shoulders, with your fingers pointing forward. Keep your elbows close to the sides of your body and rest your forehead on the floor. Relax your whole body, particularly your lower back. **❸** As you breathe in, slowly raise your head, neck and shoulders off the floor (your hips should remain firmly on the floor). Breathe out and slowly lower your body back to the starting position with your head facing in the other direction. Repeat this sequence up to 5 times.

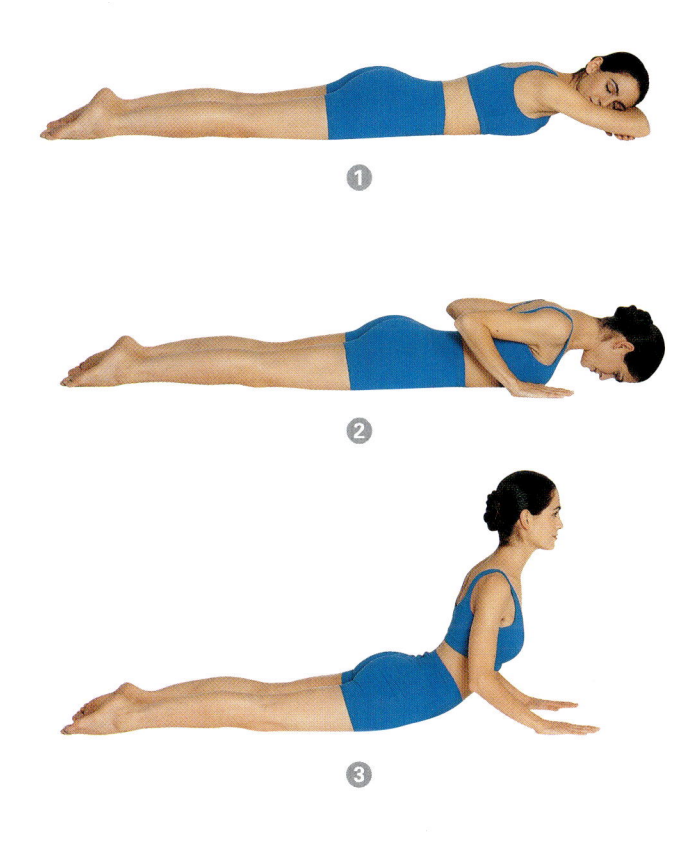

The Cobra strengthens the abdominal and back muscles and is beneficial for lower-back problems. It can also ease gynaecological problems and, because it works on the abdominal organs, it aids digestion. It is a wonderful posture for activating energy from the base chakra (*muladhara*) to the third-eye chakra (*ajna*).

People with ulcers, hernias or intestinal problems should not practise this asana without expert guidance.

The thunderbolt
vajrasana

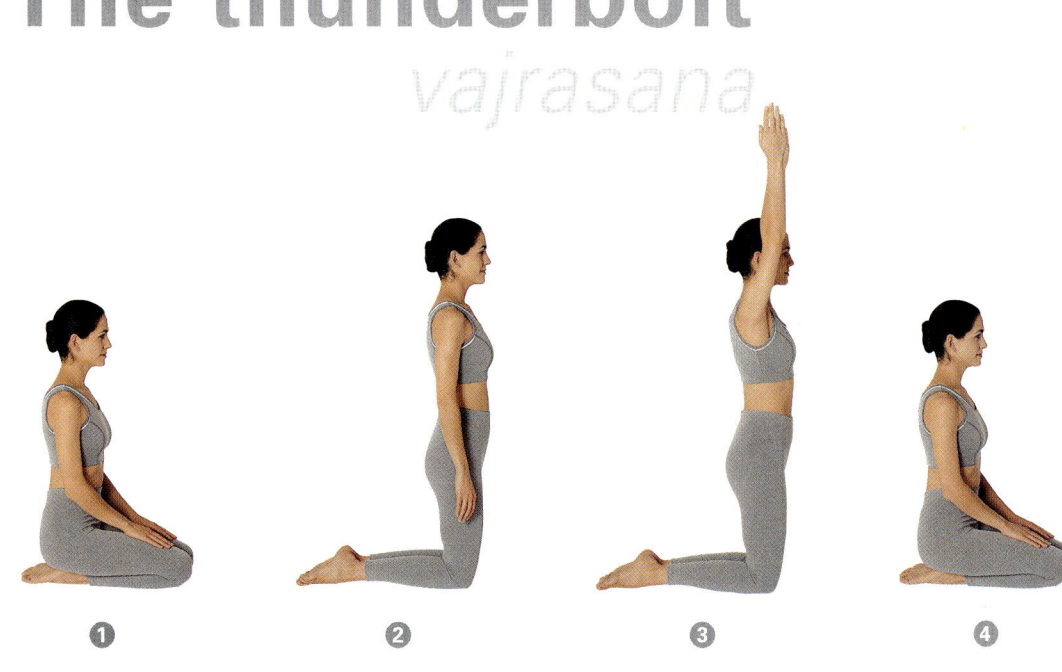

① ② ③ ④

Sitting back on your heels is a wonderful meditation posture for people who cannot sit cross-legged (even those with sciatica) and it activates life-force energy, or *prana*.

If you have varicose veins or poor circulation in the legs, place a cushion between your heels and buttocks to relieve pressure when you sit back on your heels. You may also find it helpful to put a cushion between the floor and your feet.

❶ Sit back on your heels. Your insteps should be on the floor and your big toes should be touching, with the inside edges of your feet close together. Rest your hands palms down on your knees. Make sure that your spine is straight. ❷ As you breathe in, come up from sitting into a kneeling position. Now breathe out. ❸ As you breathe in, raise your arms in an arc in front of you, bringing your hands above your head, palms facing each other. Lower your arms in an arc as you breathe out. ❹ Breathe in. Sit back on your heels as you breathe out. Repeat this sequence up to 5 times.

The butterfly
poorna titali

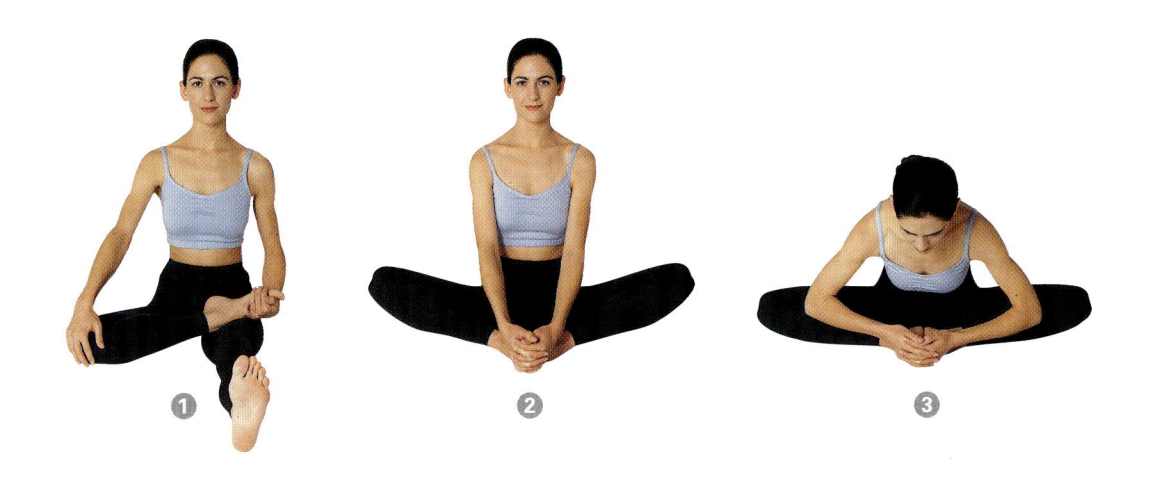

① ② ③

This is a good preparation for the Lotus posture and for sitting in meditation. The Butterfly posture relieves inner-thigh tension and is helpful if you sit or stand for long periods.

It is said that the effect created by the movement of a butterfly's wings in one part of the world can trigger a tornado thousands of miles away. So be gentle in your practice!

❶ Sit on the floor with your left leg extended. Rest your right foot on your left thigh, holding your toes with your left hand. Gently clasp your right knee with your right hand. Breathe in and out, raising and lowering your knee several times. Change legs and repeat. ❷ Bend both knees and bring the soles of the feet together. Clasp your toes. Slide your heels toward your body. Straighten your spine and breathe in. Breathe out and lower your knees to the floor. Concentrate on counting your breaths and relaxing into the posture. ❸ Bend your elbows and, working from the lower back, lower your body so that your chest comes toward the floor. Breathe in. Sit upright.

Easy spinal twist
sukhasana matsyendrasana

❶ Sit with your legs crossed at the ankles, your back straight and your palms on your knees. **❷** Breathing in deeply, raise your arms out to the sides. **❸** Rest your right palm on your left knee. Breathe out. Turn your left palm to face backward. **❹** Swing your left arm behind you and rest your palm or fingertips on the floor. Use this arm to help keep your spine straight and upright. **❺** Breathing out, gradually turn your body to the left, feeling energy moving up the spine as you do so. Look over your left shoulder. Breathe in and out. Slowly release the posture as you breathe out. Return to Step 1 and repeat the sequence, twisting to the right.

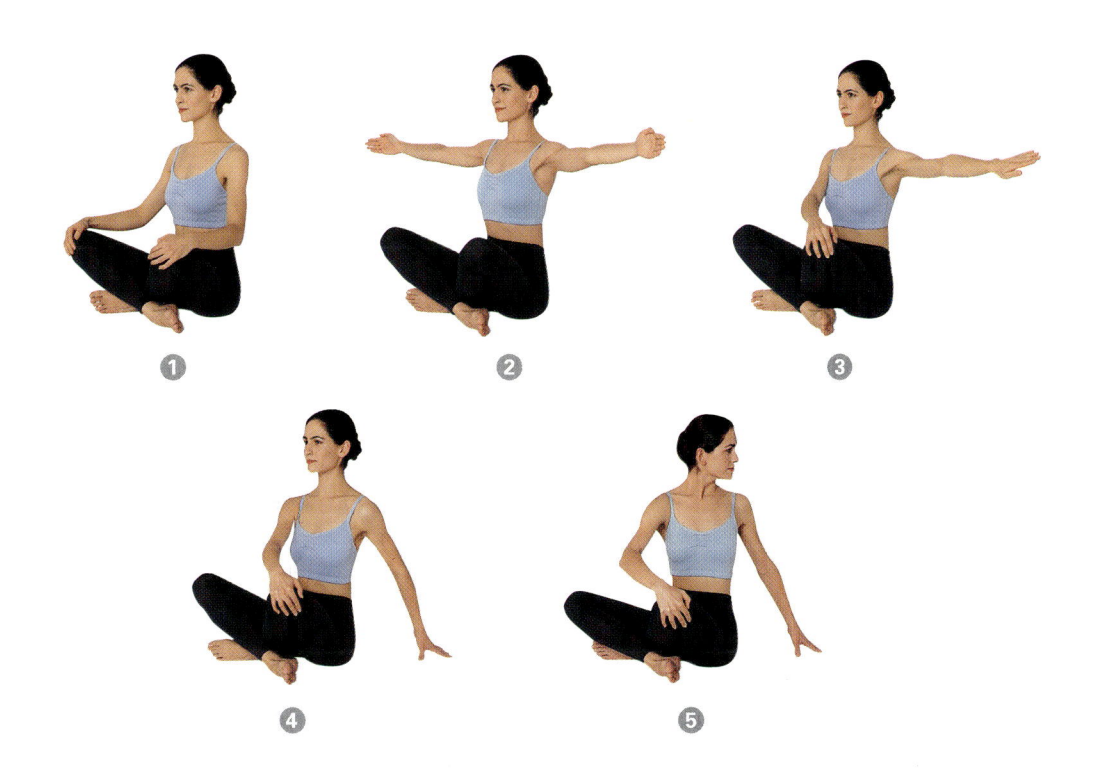

Twisting postures give the spine a wonderful workout, releasing enormous amounts of tension and flooding the spinal nerves with nutrients and energy. They open the heart chakra (*anahata*) and help to bring a greater volume of air into the lungs. They have a strong influence on the abdominal muscles as they stretch and compress them.

If you find it difficult to sit cross-legged on the floor, you can sit on a folded blanket or a firm cushion. Be careful not to over-extend yourself and twist more than your natural flexibility will permit.

The half-moon
ardha chandrasana

❶ Stand with your feet slightly apart, breathe in and raise your arms above your head. Clasp your elbows. **❷** Breathe out and bend forward at your waist, bending your knees if necessary. **❸** Place your hands on the floor. Step your right foot back, keeping your heel off the floor. **❹** Lower your right knee to the floor and straighten your toes. Breathe out. **❺** Swing your arms forward and above your head. Keep your elbows straight and palms facing. Breathe in. Sink into your hips. Focus on your breathing. **❻** Lower your palms to the floor and straighten both legs. Breathe out. **❼** Swing your right foot forward and stand up. Repeat on the other side.

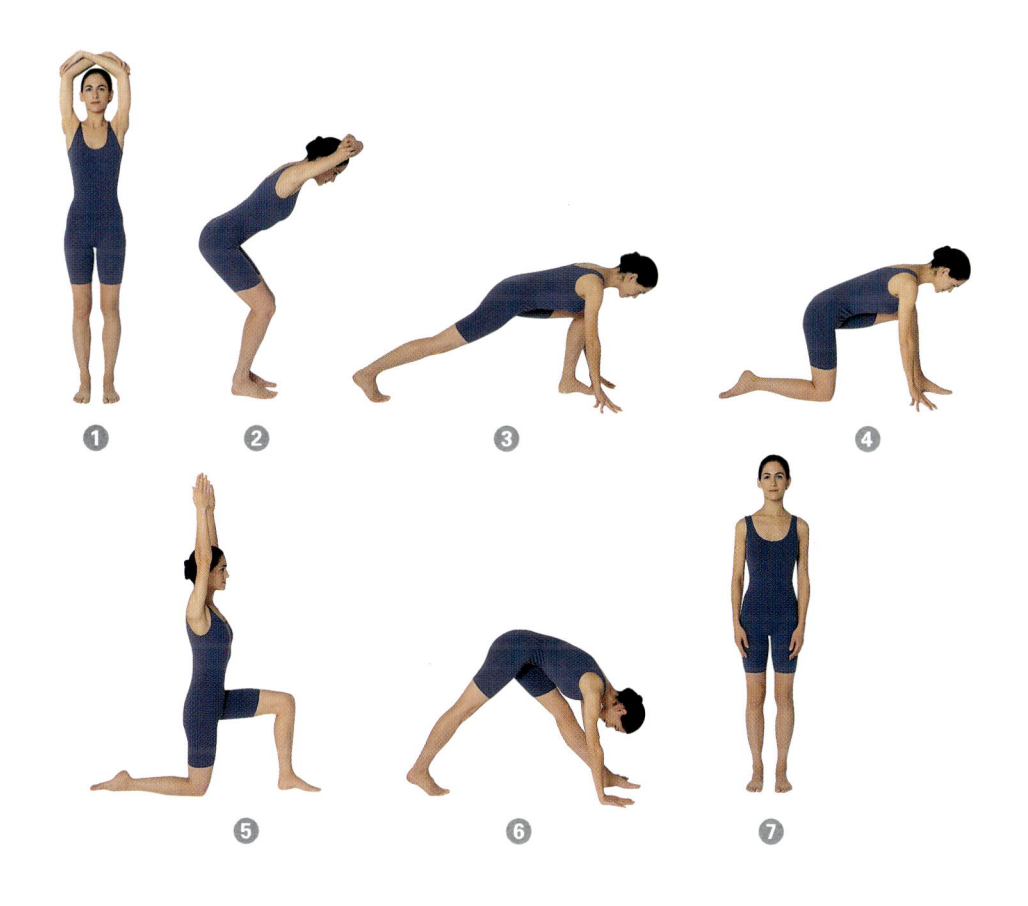

The Half-moon posture opens out the front of the chest and stretches the lungs. It strengthens the entire skeletal structure and, because it works strongly on the chest and neck, it frequently relieves respiratory ailments, including sore throats, coughs and colds. All in all it is a very invigorating posture!

When you practise this posture, focus on the sacral chakra (swadhisthana) **and on controlled movement and balance.**

The archer
akarana dhanurasana

❶ Stand with your feet hips' width apart. **❷** Step your left foot forward by a leg length and turn in your right foot so the instep aligns with your left heel. **❸** Turn your hips and upper body to the right. Raise your arms sideways to shoulder height. **❹** Look along both arms – check that they are level with your shoulders. Extend your fingers. **❺** Fold your right arm in toward your chest with your elbow at shoulder height, as if holding the string of a bow. Look along your left arm. Breathe in and out in the posture for as long as you can remain steady. Repeat on the other side.

① ② ③ ④ ⑤

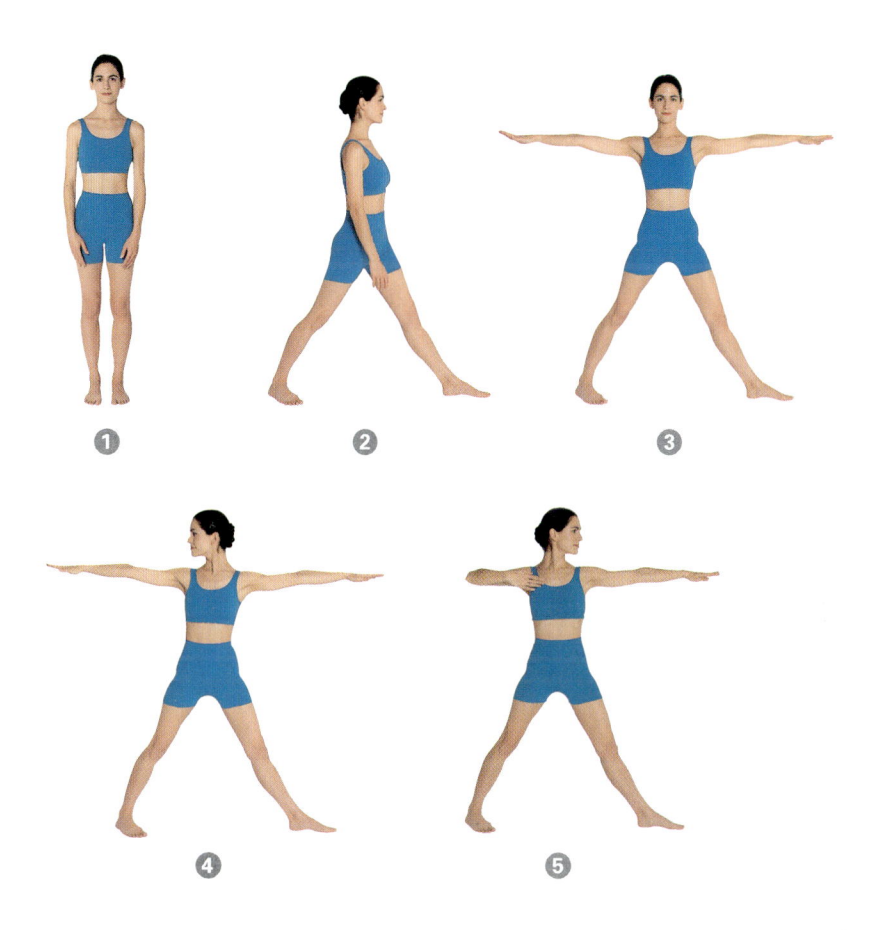

This posture works on the short, deep muscles in the neck and shoulders and is excellent for releasing tension. To enhance tension release, try sliding the bent arm forward as you breathe out and bring it back as you breathe in.

Lord Krishna advised the warrior Arjuna to learn the wisdom of skill in action: "By this I mean perfect balance, unshakeable equanimity, poise and peace of mind." *Bhagavad Gita* (2:50)

The bridge
kandharasana

1 Lie flat on your back with your arms near your sides and your palms facing down. Tilt your head slightly so that your chin moves toward your throat and the back of your neck lengthens. **2** Bend your knees and put the soles of your feet flat on the floor (first the left foot and then the right). Your feet and knees should be hips' width apart and your feet should be parallel. **3** Press down on your palms and, as you breathe in, raise your hips off the floor. Hold the posture. Breathe. Raise your hips a little more on each in-breath. **4** Breathe out and lower your hips. Stretch out your legs and then return to rest in the starting position. Repeat up to 5 times.

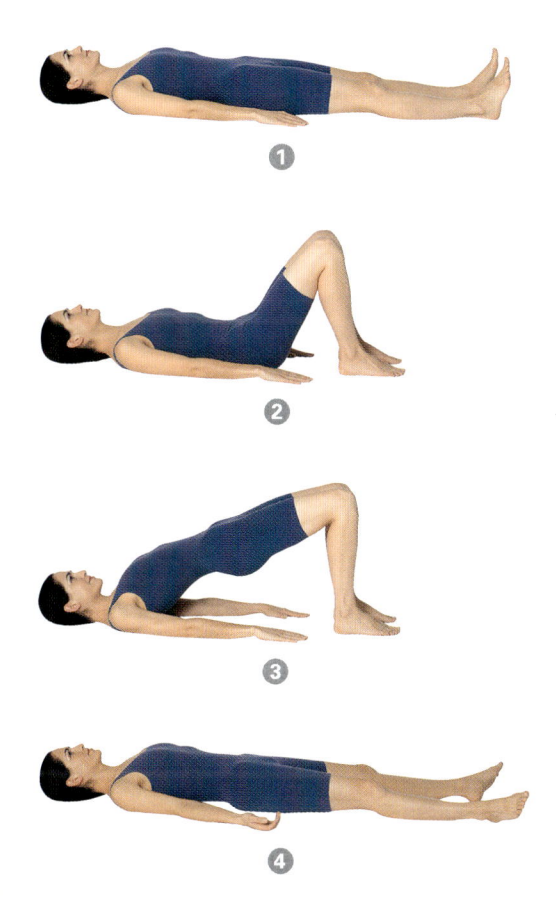

This posture massages the abdominal and female reproductive organs, improving digestion and easing menstrual problems. It can also help to realign the spine and relieve backache. People with ulcers or hernias and women in late pregnancy should avoid this posture or seek expert guidance.

When you practise this posture, focus on the heart chakra (anahata) **or the throat chakra** (vishuddhi)**.**

The plank
setu asana

❶ Sit on the floor with your legs extended, your spine straight and your hands at your sides just behind your hips. **❷** Breathe in and lift your chest, gently arching your back. Breathing out, sit upright. **❸** Take your hands a little further behind you so that your upper body is at about 45° to the floor. Keep your arms straight. **❹** Breathe in, roll your shoulders back and allow your chest to rise and your hips to lift off the floor. Gently point your toes, relax your neck and look up. Breathe. Try to raise your hips a little more on each in-breath. **❺** Breathe out and lower your hips. **❻** Gently lie down with your legs bent and your arms away from your sides. Relax.

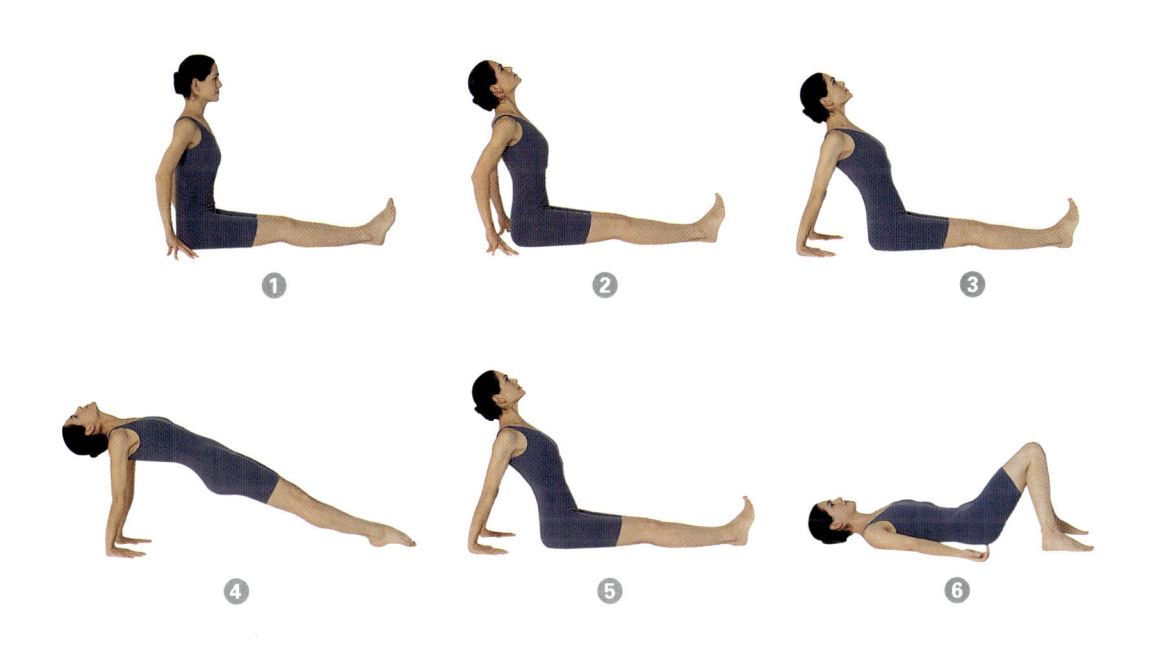

The Plank strengthens the arms, legs and the lumbar region of the spine. It is a good counterpose to forward-bending postures. You should avoid it, however, if you have high blood pressure, heart problems or a stomach ulcer. Focus on the solar-plexus chakra (*manipura*) during your practice.

When you can hold this posture comfortably, try lifting your pelvic area higher into the air. You can also try it with your hands facing backward and even lifting one arm or leg off the ground. Have fun!

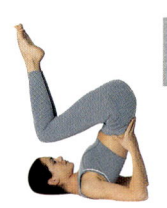

Half-shoulder stand
vipareeta karani

① Lie on your back, arms at your sides, palms facing down. ② Slide your feet toward your buttocks with your soles flat on the floor. ③ Push down with your hands and use your abdominal muscles to raise your knees. ④ Raise your legs and hips. Support your lower back with your hands. Your legs should be at a 45° angle to the floor, your feet relaxed and your elbows close together. Hold the posture and breathe. ⑤ Bring your knees to your chest, put your hands on the floor for support and slowly roll out of the pose, one vertebra at a time. ⑥ Lie down with your feet apart and your arms by your sides, palms facing up. Relax your body and breathe.

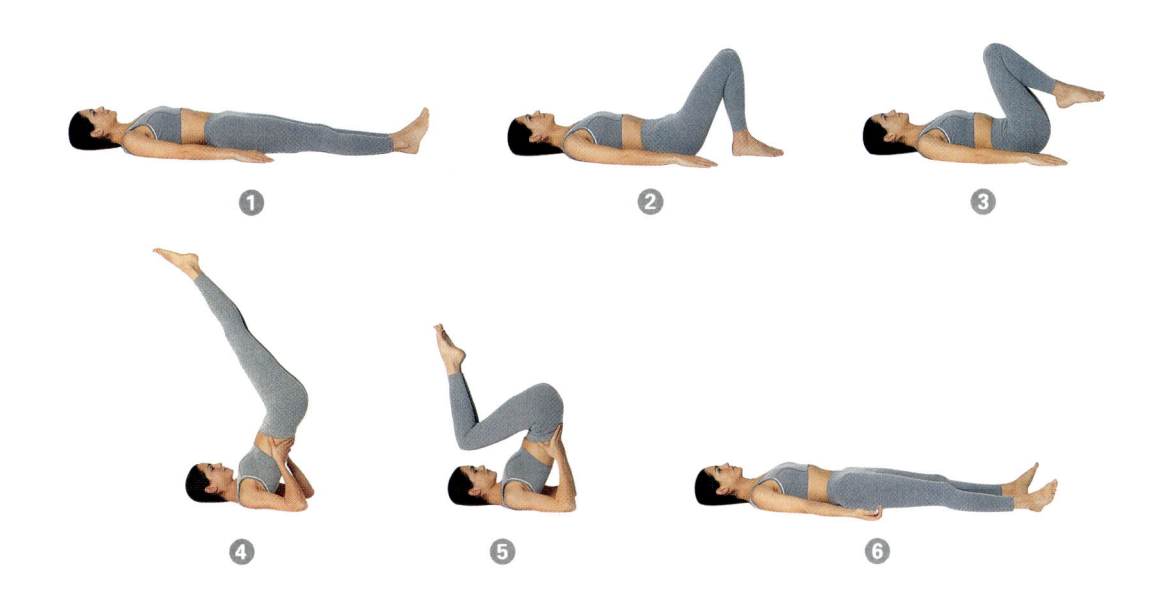

This posture stimulates the thyroid gland, relieves headaches and helps to calm mental and emotional disturbance. Do not practise it if you suffer from high blood pressure, weak blood vessels in the eyes or heart complaints. It should also be avoided during menstruation and the final stages of pregnancy.

"One achieves serenity by focusing on the inner light." *Yoga Sutras of Patanjali* (1:36)

The fish
matsyasana

① Sit on the floor, legs extended, spine upright and hands behind your hips. ② Breathing out, lower yourself to the floor using your forearms for support. ③ Slide your hands toward your feet. Raise your chest and rest the back of your head on the floor. Keep your chest raised as high as possible. Breathe in and out for as long as you are comfortable. ④ To release, slide your hands under your lower back, press down on your hands and elbows and lift your head. ⑤ Lie down. Release your hands, link your fingers and cradle your head in your hands. Pull your knees toward your chest. Cross your ankles and let your knees drop. Relax totally and focus on your breath.

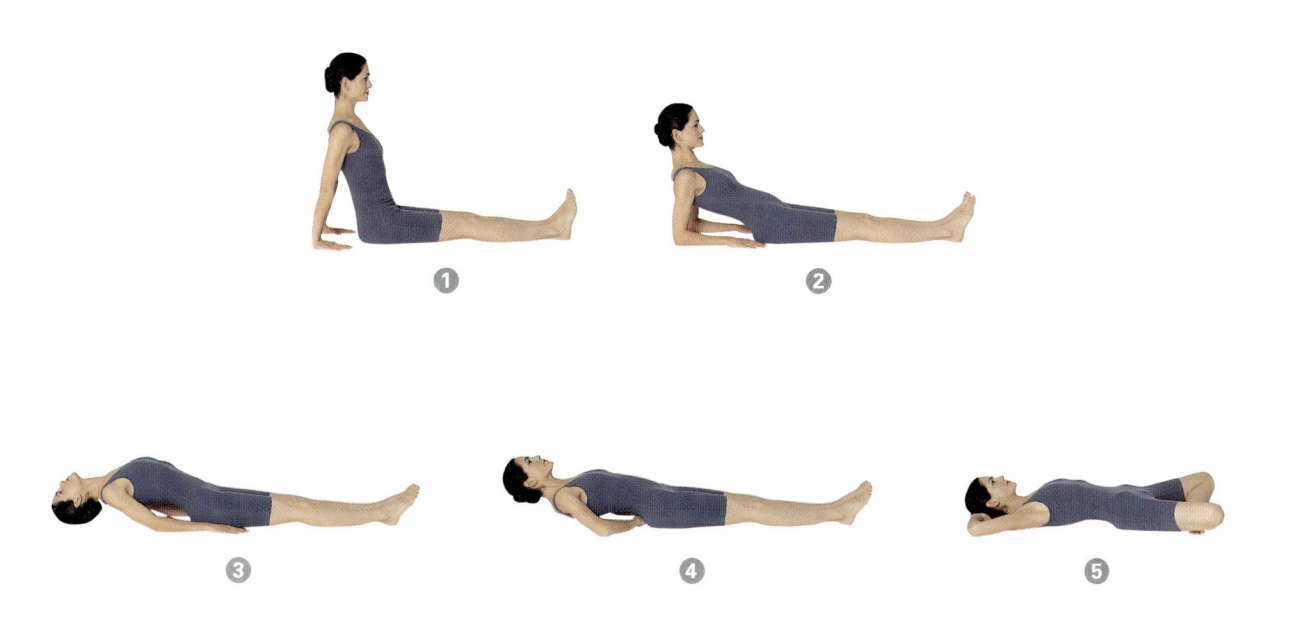

This posture opens up the chest and neck and is useful for abdominal and respiratory complaints, including colds and 'flu. It is also a very energizing posture. Take care getting in and out of this posture and avoid it altogether if you are pregnant, or suffer from heart disease or other serious health problems.

When you practise this posture, focus on the heart chakra (anahata) **in Step 3 and on the solar-plexus chakra** (manipura) **for the final relaxation.**

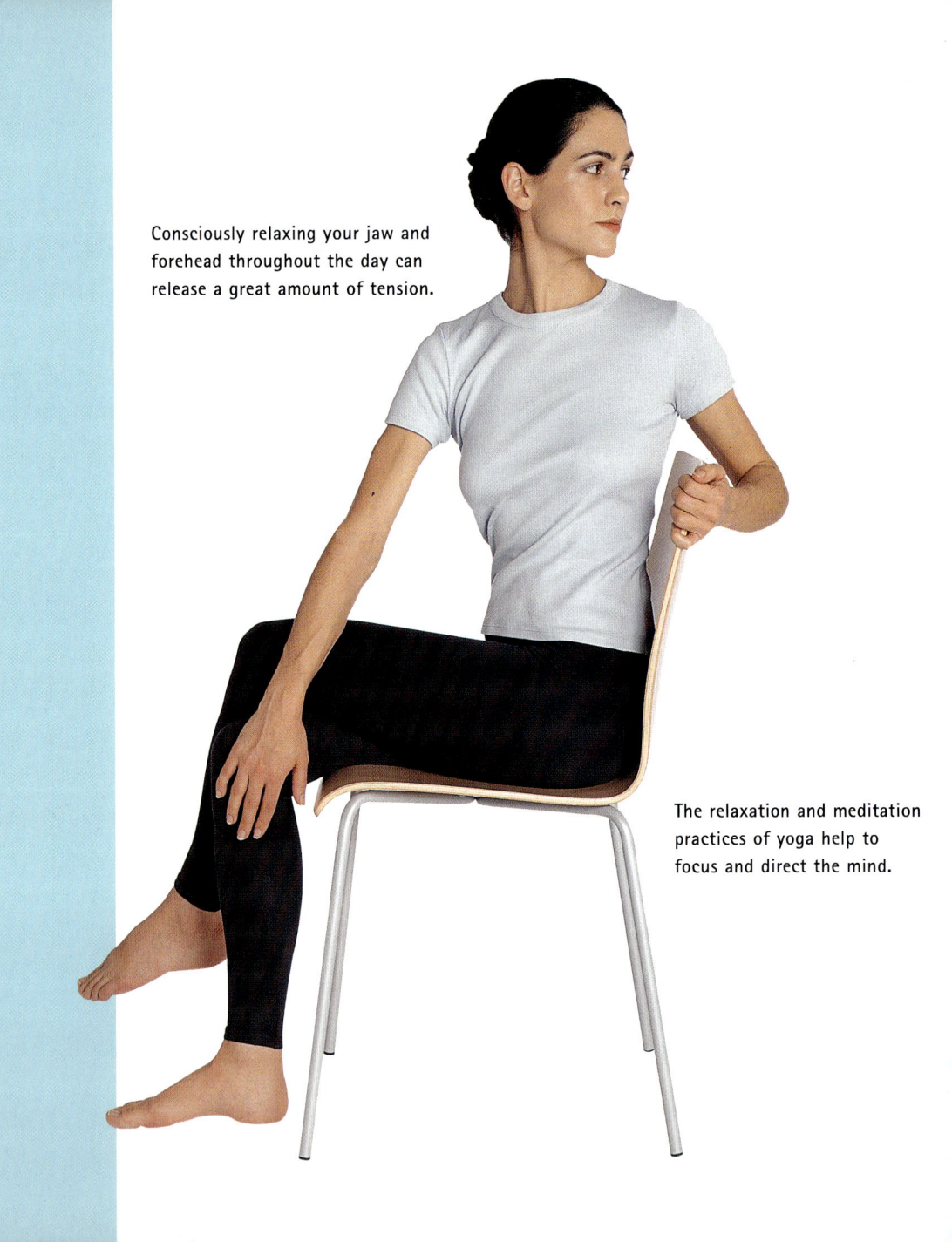

Consciously relaxing your jaw and forehead throughout the day can release a great amount of tension.

The relaxation and meditation practices of yoga help to focus and direct the mind.

chapter four
Yoga all day

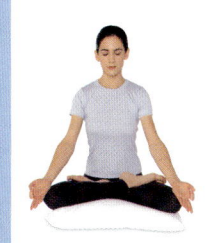

Yoga is a discipline that, when incorporated into your everyday life, will have a profoundly beneficial effect.

In this chapter are modifications to the classic postures, designed specifically for use during the day, at home or at work. They can be practised without any special preparation, and will enhance your energy levels and make your day flow smoothly. They will also help to relieve fatigue, muscle tension and stress.

Our waking lives are often dominated by mental chatter or uncontrolled and chaotic thoughts. By being mindful of our breathing we can learn to still this internal dialogue and approach situations and people as calmly as possible.

Morning stretch
revitalize your body

① Stand up straight with your hands in the prayer position. **②** Breathing in, raise your arms in an arc above your head, fold your arms and clasp your elbows. Breathing out, bend forward at the hips. Extend your spine. **③** Lower your hands to the floor. **④** Step your feet back (right then left). Lift your hips up high and drop your heels to the floor. **⑤** Breathe out and bring your knees to the floor. Breathe in, raise your head, tilt your hips and let your spine hollow. **⑥** Breathe out, lift your abdomen, lower your head and look between your legs. Repeat Steps 5 and 6 twice. **⑦** Push back, sit on your heels and stretch from your fingertips to the base of your spine. **⑧** Sit upright. Put your palms on your knees. Focus on your breathing.

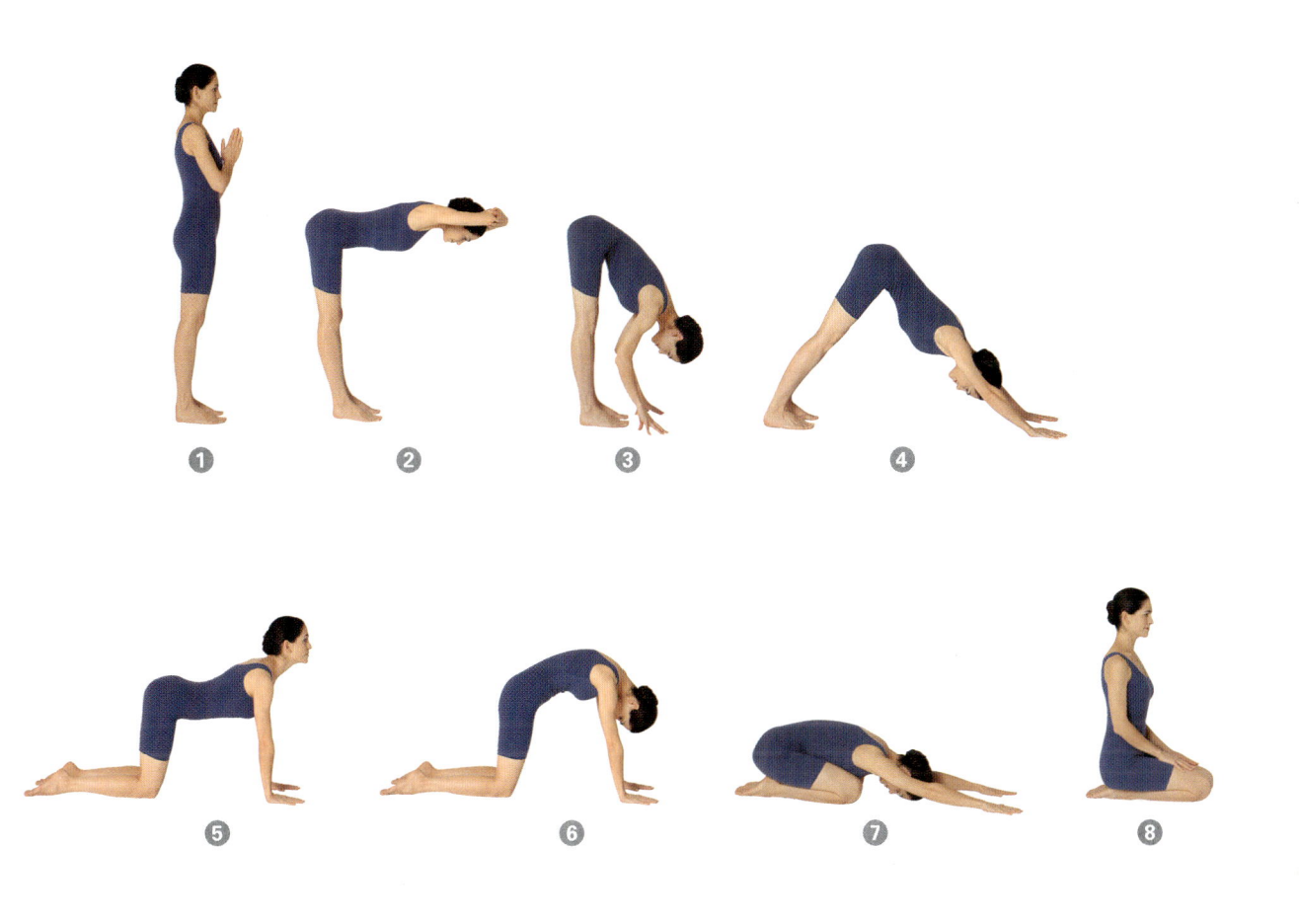

Give yourself at least 10 or 15 minutes for this sequence – it will invigorate you, balance your energy and prepare you for the day.

In the final stage of this sequence, close your eyes and make a resolution for the day. Open your eyes and smile.

Yoga at work

5 fast energy boosters

Forward extension

Spinal twist

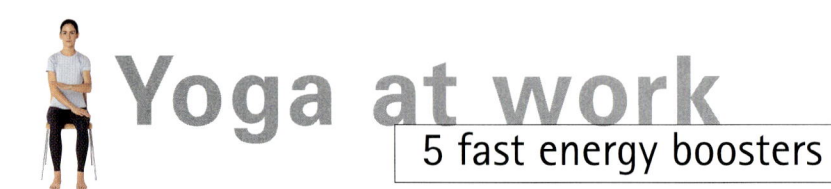

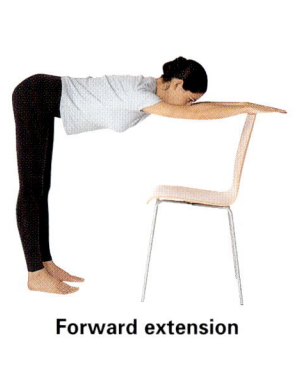

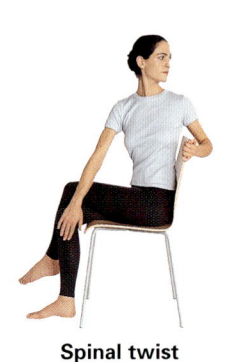

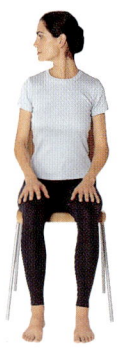

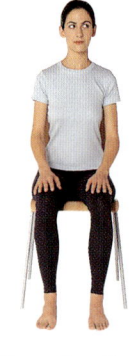

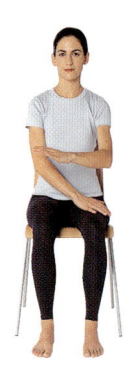

Head rotation

Eye relaxation

Cross crawl

When you start to run out of energy at work or at home during the day, these simple yoga practices can be invaluable.

These postures are even more effective if you concentrate on your breath and allow your mind to clear.

Forward extension Stand facing a chair. Bend and hold the back of the chair so that your legs are at 90° to your body. Elongate your spine and stretch your fingers.

Spinal twist Sit upright and cross your left leg over your right. Put your right hand over your left knee, your left hand on the chair back. Lift up your spine and twist your body to the left. Repeat on the other side.

Head rotation Sit or stand. Breathing out, turn your head to the right. Breathing in, return to centre. Breathing out, turn to the left. Do this for 2 minutes.

Eye relaxation Imagine a clock face around your eyes. Look at 12 o'clock and count each numeral clockwise. Now do this counter-clockwise. Repeat several times.

Cross crawl Cross your arms and simply tap each knee in turn. Try to synchronize your breathing with the taps.

Evening practice

centre yourself after the day

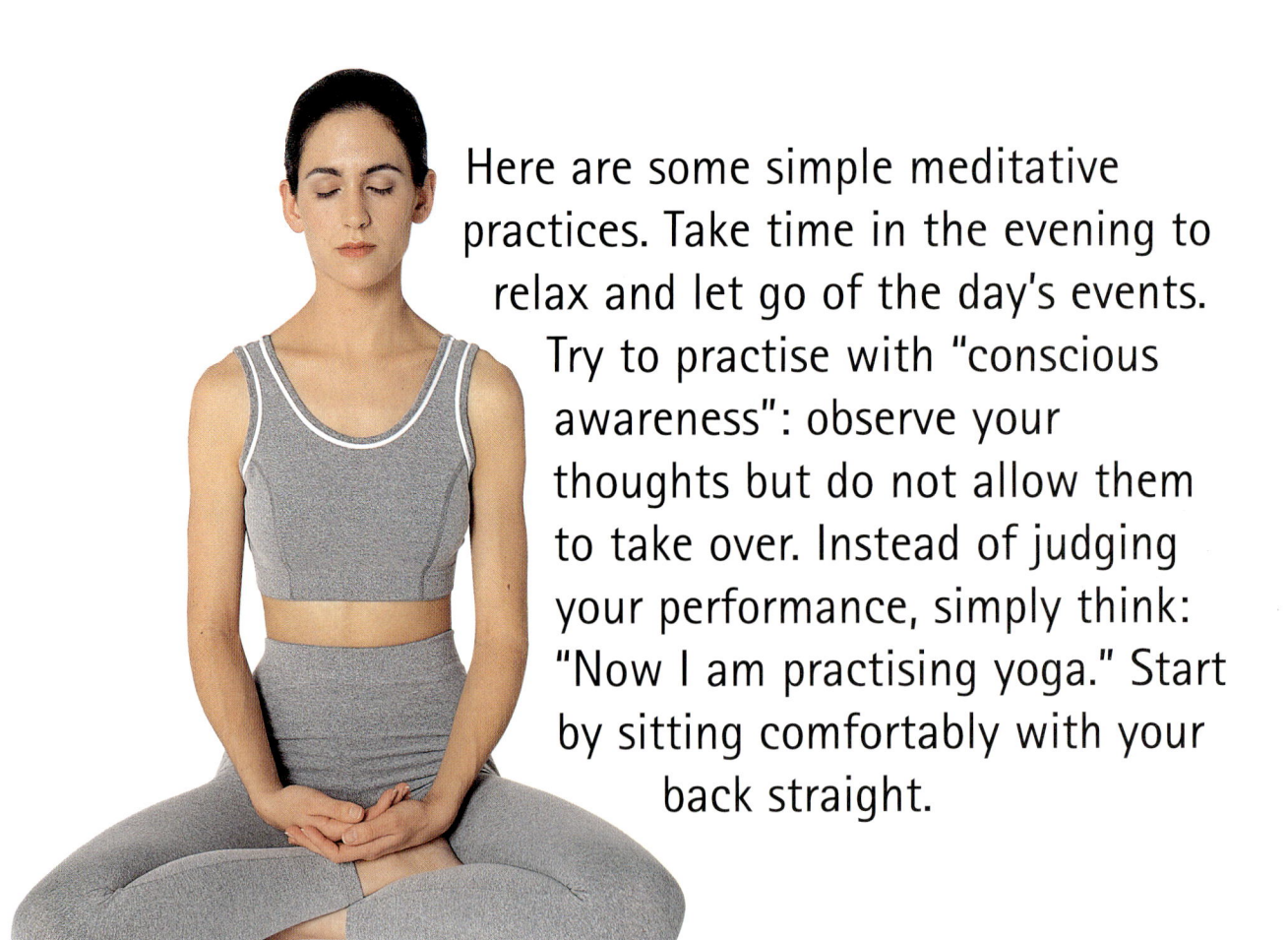

Here are some simple meditative practices. Take time in the evening to relax and let go of the day's events. Try to practise with "conscious awareness": observe your thoughts but do not allow them to take over. Instead of judging your performance, simply think: "Now I am practising yoga." Start by sitting comfortably with your back straight.

Humming-bee practice Close your eyes and relax. Close the flaps of your ears with your index fingers. Imagine a humming bee inside your head. Breathe in. Breathe out and make the even, controlled noise of a humming bee. Repeat up to 5 times. This produces a meditational state and eases stress and insomnia.

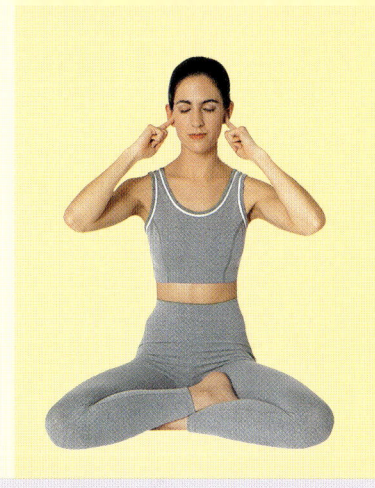

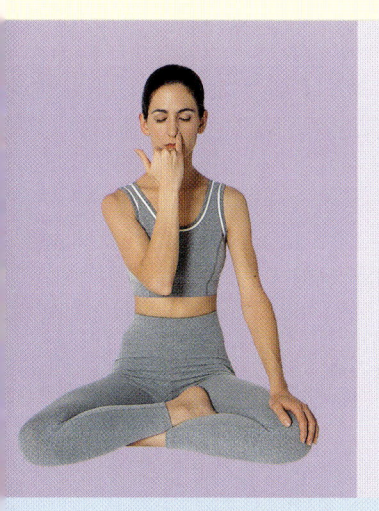

Alternate-nostril breathing Hold the right nostril closed with the thumb and breathe into the left nostril. Close the left nostril with the little finger, release the right nostril and breathe out. Breathe in through the right nostril, then close it with your thumb. Release your left nostril and breathe out. Repeat several times.

Visualization of chakras and colours Imagine drawing up red-coloured energy from the earth into your base chakra. Visualize the colour changes (red, orange, yellow, green, blue and violet) as the energy ascends the differently coloured chakras. At the crown chakra the energy becomes white, creating an envelope around you.

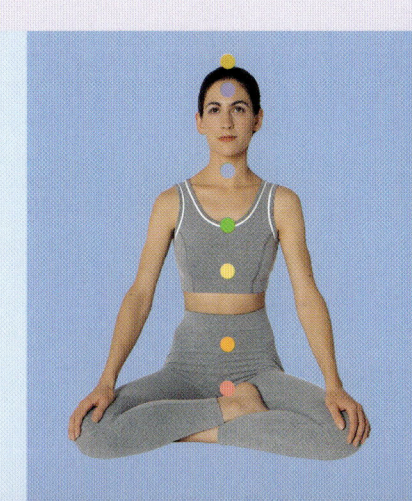

Bedtime relaxation
preparation for sleep

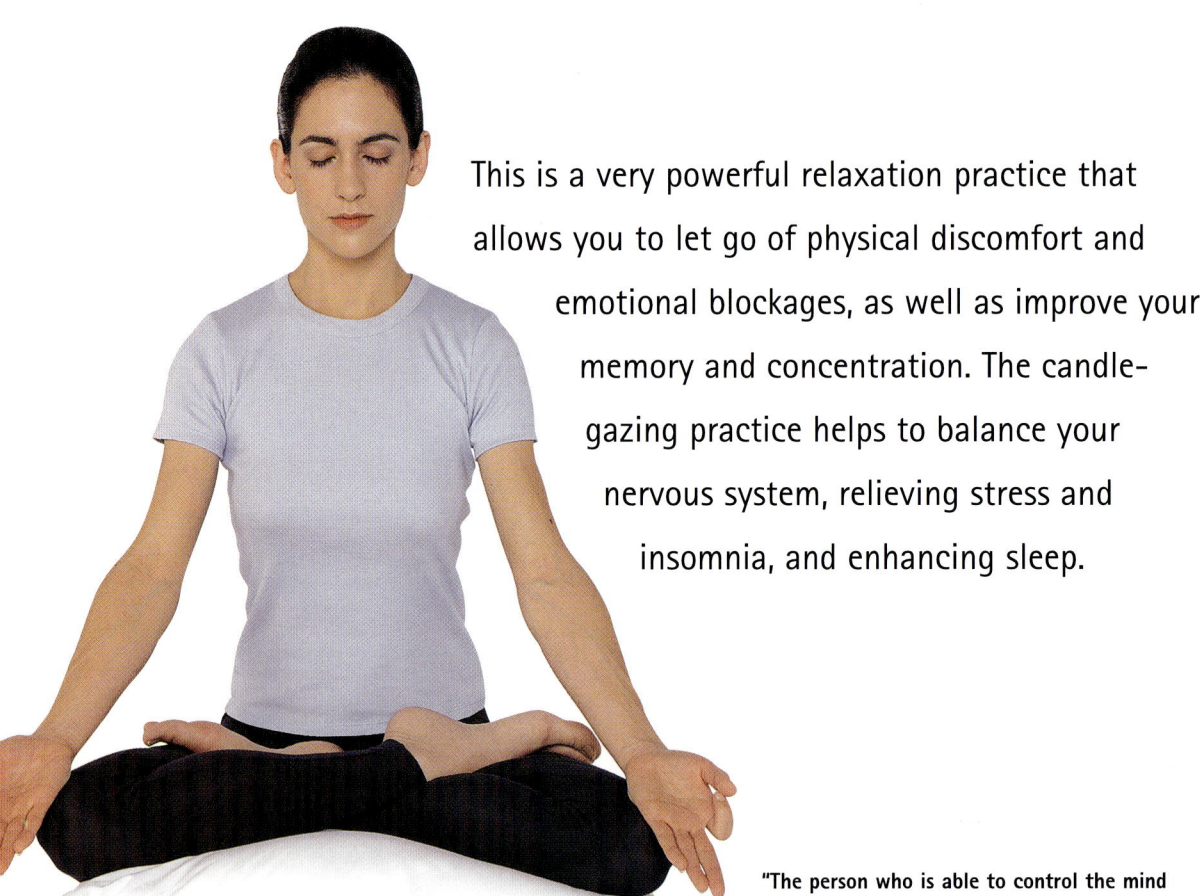

This is a very powerful relaxation practice that allows you to let go of physical discomfort and emotional blockages, as well as improve your memory and concentration. The candle-gazing practice helps to balance your nervous system, relieving stress and insomnia, and enhancing sleep.

"The person who is able to control the mind and engage in actions without attachment is able to excel." *Bhagavad Gita* (3:7)

Light a candle and your favourite incense. Spend a few minutes thinking over the events of the day and then let go of these thoughts. Make an agreement with yourself that for the next 15–20 minutes your thoughts will be on the practice of relaxation and meditation. Sit in a comfortable position with your back straight. Spend some minutes looking at the candle flame. Close your eyes and hold the image in your mind. When the image disappears, open your eyes and look at the flame again. Repeat this a few times.

Remain sitting or lie down on the floor in the relaxation pose, *shavasana* (see pp.18–19), but do not fall asleep. Practise yoga breathing (see pp.24–25) or alternate-nostril breathing (see p.69) for a few minutes and then scan your body, looking for tension. Breathe into any areas of tension and, when you breathe out, allow them to soften and release.

Now visualize the candle flame on the screen of your mind. Allow it to be small at first but, as you watch, see it grow bigger and brighter, washing over your body, bringing peace, love and compassion. Allow the flame to fill every aspect of your interior space and then let it focus at the heart chakra (*anahata*).

Allow this image to fade and bring your awareness to the breath at the tip of your nose. Then gradually become aware of your body, starting with your fingers and toes. When you are ready, gently open your eyes.

Index

A
abdomen
  complaints 61
  massage 55
  muscle strengthening 43, 49
Archer posture (*akarana dhanurasana*) 52-3
arm stretches (*tiryaka tadasana*) 30-31
arms, strengthening of 37, 57
asana see posture

B
back muscles 33, 39, 41, 43
back problems 19, 33, 43, 55
Bhakti yoga 10
breathing (*pranayama*) 10-11, 24-5
  awareness and 19, 21, 23, 24, 71
  contact with *purusa* 15
  meditative practice and 69, 71
  stilling internal dialogue 63
Bridge posture (*kandharasana*) 54-5
Butterfly posture (*poorna titali*) 46-7

C
candle gazing 70-71
Cat posture (*marjari-asana*) 34-5
chakras 12-13
  Bridge posture and 55
  Cat posture and 34
  Cobra exercise and 43
  Downward-facing dog and 37
  Fish exercise and 61
  Half-moon posture and 51
  Leg lift posture and 41
  Plank posture and 57
  twisting postures and 49
  visualization and 69, 71
child, pose of the (*supta shashankasana*) 38-9
circulation 34, 37, 44
cleansing (*shatkarmas*) 10-11
Cobra posture (*bhujangasana*) 42-3
concentration 41, 70
consciousness 9
Corpse pose (*shavasana*) 18-19, 71
Cross crawl 66-7

D
dhyana see meditation
digestion and digestive tract 34, 43, 55
Downward-facing dog (*adho mukha shvanasana*) 36-7

E
emotional problems 59, 70
energy (*prana*)
  activation of 44
  balance 12-13, 65
  boosters 66-7
  building up energy levels 33
  flow of 12-13, 29-61
everyday yoga 62-71
eye relaxation 66-7

F
Fish posture (*matsyasana*) 60-61
Forward bend (*utthanasana*) 32-3
Forward extension 66-7

G
gynaecological problems 43

H
Half-shoulder stand (*vipareeta karani*) 58-9
Half-moon posture (*ardha chandrasana*) 50-51
Hatha yoga 10
Hatha Yoga Pradipika 11
head rotation 66-7
headaches 59
Humming-bee meditation 69

J
Jnana yoga 10

K
Karma yoga 10
kriyas see cleansing

L
Leg lift (*ardha shalabhasana*) 40-41
legs
  inner thigh tension 46
  strengthening of 37, 57
life-force energy *see* energy
Lotus posture, preparation for 46-7

M
meditation (*dhyana*) 10-11, 71
  postures 44-5, 46-7, 68-9
menstrual problems 34, 55
mental disturbance 59
Mountain pose (*tadasana*) 22-3

N
nadis 12-13
neck muscles 53

P
paths of yoga 10-11
pawanmuktasanas see warm-ups
Plank posture (*setu asana*) 56-7
posture (*asana*) 10-11, 13, 17-27, 29-61
prana see energy
pranayama see breathing
purusa, making contact with 15

R
Raja yoga 10
relaxation
  eye relaxation 66-7
  postures 18-19, 38-9, 70-71
reproductive organs 55
respiratory ailments 51, 61

S
self
  centring 18-19
  preparation 17-27
shatkarmas see cleansing
shoulder muscles 53
sitting postures 20-21, 25, 26-7, 44-9, 56-7, 66-71
skeletal structure, strengthening of 51
Spinal twist (*sukhasana matsyendrasana*) 48-9, 66-7
spine 34, 37, 39, 49, 55, 57
Staff pose (*dandasana*) 20-21
standing postures 22-3, 30-33
stillness *see purusa*
stress management 14, 29
  see also tension
stretching 30-31, 39, 64-5

T
tension
  release of 22-3, 49, 53, 62, 71
  see also stress
Thunderbolt posture (*vajrasana*) 44-5
thyroid gland stimulation 59
twisting postures 48-9, 66-7

V
varicose veins 44
visualization 69
vital force *see* energy

W
warm-ups (*pawanmuktasanas*) 26-7

ACKNOWLEDGMENTS

The Publishers would like to thank model Tara Fraser, and make-up artist/hairdresser Elizabeth Lawson.